Foreword

I was away on holiday in Britain when a g happened to me. I was trying to climb some stairs and my right leg refused to function. I said nothing to my partner, Douglas. I suffered from rheumatoid arthritis and wondered if it was simply a flare-up and would right itself. I decided to push this incident to the back of my mind and cope as well as I could. It was nothing major. But then my ribcage began to hurt. I could not get comfortable at night. I ceased to sleep. I took over-the-counter medication and silently began to count down the days till I returned home.

Back in Napier I rang my doctor. The receptionist asked me if my case was urgent. She explained to me the doctor was busy with an outbreak of the flu. I thought for a moment and said 'No.' (Were my complaints urgent? I wasn't sure.) She directed me to a 24/7 medical practice.

On my third visit I came across my own doctor twilighting, and she agreed to see me. Only at the last moment did she order a PSA test. When it came back she sat me down and said, 'I have some bad news, Peter. You have prostate cancer and it is in your bones. It has been left too late to do anything.' She did not say specifically, 'And you will die.' Perhaps she didn't need to.

In Auckland a close friend managed to get me into a cancer specialist at short notice. The radiologist, who had stayed behind late to see me, wanted me to go into hospital that night. I replied I could not – 'I need to go home and collect my stuff.' (I meant pyjamas, toothpaste, a book. I didn't really know what I needed. I just wanted time to slow down so I could control what was happening to me.)

The following morning I found myself in Auckland Hospital, in 'Acute Oncology', in a room with three other men. All appeared to be seriously ill. Perhaps there was a shortage of beds, I thought. In fact, I abandoned reason at this point. I had been living with incremental pain for so long, I simply accepted it as part of how things were. And so I began my sojourn in the strangest territory I had ever been in.

I was 67 years old. My mother, aged almost 101, had died six months earlier. I thought I knew where I was in life. Instead, in a state of self-deception, wracked with physical pain that was so constant I could barely discern reality, I had ended up in a ward with three other men, all of whom were on the cliff edge of dying.

This took me a day or so to work out. But in a public ward there are no secrets. So when the young father – probably not even 30 – was told there was no longer any use in chemo and he should contact the hospice for further pain management, we other three men listened to the depth of his silence, the absence of tears, the long hard shock of acceptance. By this stage I was having Sevredol, a morphine-based pain relief, every hour. This had done its work. It submerged my pain within my body – or maybe my consciousness lifted the pain out of my body and reduced it to something not only bearable but at times almost ecstatic. I was alive! I was not dying. I was alive.

I am not sure at what point I decided to post on Facebook. This was not a conscious decision. It was an inevitable decision. I was a writer. I had no pen or paper. So how could I talk to

Hello
Darkness

For Douglas

Hello
Darkness

Peter Wells

MIGHTY AJAX PRESS

First published 2019
Mighty Ajax Press
260 Great South Road, Auckland 1051
mightyajaxpress@gmail.com

ISBN 978-0-473-45162-2

A catalogue record for this book is available from
the National Library of New Zealand

Photograph on page 122 by Patricia Robb
Book design by Katrina Duncan
Cover design by Keely O'Shannessy

This book was printed on FSC certified paper

Printed in China by Everbest Printing Investment Ltd

'my world'? Through Facebook? This is an interesting concept as I am not certain I had much of an idea of who I talked with or to on FB. There were certain people like David Herkt, an author and old friend, whose erudite posts were always a pleasure to read. There were others, people whose posts I read intermittently, sometimes in a funk of boredom, an edgy wish to be entertained or at least diverted from stasis. There were people I knew by sight, by history; and then there were people who were 'acquaintances'– people you 'knew' on FB but who failed to say hello when you walked past them in the street.

I had no particular faith in FB and it was sheer luck that I had not followed close friends in their exit from a medium seen as tainted. (This was months before the Cambridge Analytica revelations, I should add.) William Yang, another friend, confessed to me that while he posted, he considered some people 'FB tragics'. Was I on the border of being a FB tragic – meaning, I think, someone whose digital life is stronger than their actual life? Whose FB presence was an act of willed ventriloquism while their physical life suffered a kind of emotional starvation?

When I did my first FB post from Ward 64 I did not let any of this enter my head. Instead I was overcome with an almost awful sense of urgency. Was it that I had news to tell: I am going to die sooner rather than later? Yes. But it was more than that. I suddenly understood that I had entered what Susan Sontag, in *Illness as Metaphor*, so memorably called 'the night side of life'. As she said, 'Everybody who is born holds dual citizenship, in the kingdom of the well and in the kingdom of the sick. Although we all prefer to use only the good passport, sooner or later each one of us is obliged to identify ourselves as citizens of that other place.'

I had become a 'citizen of that other place'. I was in a fundamentally changed landscape and one I needed to describe. Perhaps the morphine disinhibited me. But I began to do posts on FB which were, for better or worse, broadcasts from this strange new landscape.

The reaction right from the start was strong – 114 comments on my first post: part shock at my disclosure, I guess, but also something deeper – could one say it was a response to the emotional resonance of my situation? I was breaking an ordinance by being so emotional, direct and straightforward. I was not presenting information in a way that implied I wanted admiration or condoning. It was more profound – a call for help, for empathy. At the same time it was clear the posts were 'reports on experience', nothing more or less.

The response was electric and almost always in the same vein of intensity. Replies multiplied – people I did not know well responded personally. Then I did something I had never done before. I answered, I commented. Before this I had resented the stale fug of FB, but now I was not just highly keyed emotionally, I was acutely lonely. I was hungry for connection, often at unearthly hours like 3 a.m. Friends on the other side of the world got in touch. Irene Malone in Malaysia was awake when everyone in New Zealand was asleep. My brother's old boyfriend, now in Montreal, with whom I'd lost touch. In London Jonathan Denis's sister, Kirsten, said hi.

Now I seemed to live in a hurricane of comments which both helped me and pushed me forward. Constructing a daily post became my day's activity – everything was bent towards it, my thoughts, feelings, perceptions. It gave me purpose.

It didn't save my life – it was doctors and nurses and meds doing that – but posting kept me sane, located me, pivoted me. It was a stake in the ground of a self which I otherwise risked losing as everything changed around me – how I would live life, approach the future, expect to live.

Then two things happened pretty much simultaneously. Mary McCallum from Makāro Press asked me if a medical site ('Corpus: Conversations about Medicine and Life', with 421 subscribers) could republish a post I wrote praising Ronnie, the night nurse. Then Linda Burgess, an old friend, contacted Steve Braunias, literary editor of The Spinoff, alerting him to my posts. Braunias got in touch and asked me if I wanted to reprint a run of postings on The Spinoff. He would edit them into a substantial 6,000-word 'edition', and The Spinoff would publish them on line. This changed the dimension of everything.

It was as if I had punctured the surface of my privacy and been launched into a wider world. Now FB requests were a daily marathon and I no longer queried who might want to befriend me (within limits). This appeared to push the postings into a different, almost public category. They notified more people about my existence – my writing – my dilemma – and my writing became available to a wider readership.

Yet in the midst of this I did begin to wonder what I had done, was doing. Was I betraying some essence of myself by making my innermost thoughts and fears so public? Wasn't it almost a form of emotional boasting, as if showing off the excesses of my emotional state?

There must always be private spaces, even in such an open 'public' life. I accept that. But I also had a different view. What I responded to specifically was the liveliness of the medium, the way a comment could appear out of nowhere, you could reply, they could reply. In a situation of dead calm that promised only a shortened life, this luxuriance of activity, this disturbance of stillness, was invigorating. Isolated in my hospital room – or later at home – I felt fully engaged with 'life'.

The fact was I needed Facebook – just as I, to a degree, imposed my will on it. I was aware I was writing in as frank a manner as I could. Behind me lay a lifetime's diary writing. As an isolated kid, a diary had been a survival mechanism: it was how I talked to myself and it was how I reconstructed the world. There was a deliberate and clear line from those earliest diary explorations to the frank writing I did on FB: it had the intimacy of a diary, and also something else. A diary is or should be an informal truth tribunal. So if one part of my brain told me FB was an inherently corrupt and even corrupting medium, another part of my brain told me it provided a format that allowed me to speak my truth: how I was experiencing my life with prostate cancer – how, in a larger sense, I faced issues of mortality. I assumed the frankness I needed. I was open. I overlooked whatever was negative or trivial within the medium and asserted a seriousness of intent, which FB friends met in kind.

That's what made the dialogue – and I see the postings inherently as a dialogue – so enriching. I was encouraged, accompanied, associated with empathy. As I posted, so people replied. I was not alone. I can't emphasise this enough. Isolation is what makes illness so depleting. You are trapped in a prison of self – a damaged self. I never felt that. I was surrounded by voices. Nearly every post you read here was surrounded by multiple voices replying, offering advice, commentary, comparisons. These replies could occur over a day, or days. All through the night. And I have to confess the quick flutter of responses was very like being patted – as if you were a cat or a dog and this was a physical, intimate touch. You feel connected, and in a disconnected world this is good.

So in the end I ended up writing about my most private feelings in a public, open medium (Facebook), using a twenty-first-century form of communication (an iPhone), but in the form of an almost ancient literary device – a diary in which I talked about the most urgent six months of my life. In this time I strove to make sense of my situation, which seemed to alter so constantly I could never quite grasp it. Like anyone really sick, I re-thought my life. I faced my regrets – or at least some of them. (I'm 68 now – I have a lot of regrets.) I talked about intimate things – sleeplessness, fears of losing my masculinity, the beauty of friendship, the loveliness of ordinary human courtesies. The entries were essentially daily bulletins. I spent a lot of time formulating them. It's not too much to say they shaped my day (and for this I am intensely grateful – the invalid's worst enemy is long unshaped undifferentiated time). Often a small fragment would occur to me in the morning. From that would spring a cluster of thoughts. Once they were clear in pattern I sat down with my iPhone and began writing. In hospital, it was all I had. Besides, I discovered a liking for the smallness of the screen: as a child I had written my diaries in the tiniest handwriting, evading the glance of adults. Once I was happy with the piece, I emailed it to my computer (to look at again when I came home). There I did the fine editing and posted it, usually in the early hours of the morning. I kept to these two things throughout, composing on my iPhone and posting in the early hours. They were my strange good luck tokens – the things that made me who I was. They took me back too to the knife edge of crisis: they reminded me of where I had come from.

This book, then, is the story of six months in my life, told in diary segments that accrue over time the weight and logic, I hope, of a narrative, building up in momentum so that, though fragmentary, they yet form a whole: an intimate picture of a person who goes through life-changing events and comes out the other side. But this book is not merely the sum of the original FB posts and The Spinoff version so ably edited by Steve Braunias. I have added in private diary musings I did not put up on FB. Why not? Things were happening so fast I wanted to slow down my life into the stillness of intro-spection. Some things I needed to hide. The outcome of these changes is that *Hello Darkness* is the new, definitive version of my writing at that time. Luckily, I have been able to put this book together from a position of strength and relative health. I see the whole now as I didn't see it at the time. And the surprising thing to me is that I have produced not only a record of my time in extremis but also what amounts to a companion piece to my 2017 family memoir, *Dear Oliver*: naked autobiography you could call it.

All along I wanted to keep speaking, as it were, one to one. The intimacy to me is very important – the aspect of a conversation. Hence why the book is called *Hello Darkness*, after the old Simon and Garfunkel song. A really important if unsaid part is the well-known refrain. From this I take the lovely familiarity of old friends coming together to exchange thoughts, trusting in one another, even if they have not spoken for a long time. My wish is the reader feels the same.

Hello Darkness

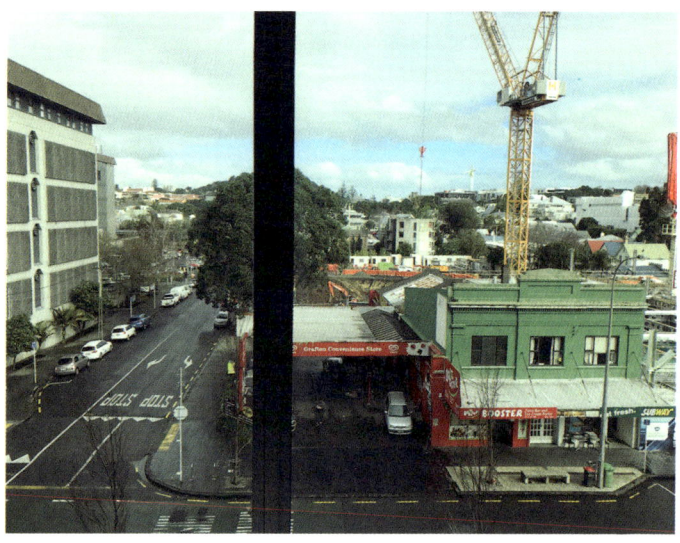

November 15, 10.45 a.m.

View from my hospital room. In the foreground, the green building is where I flatted with my brother Russell in 1974. Russell was a great stylist and the flat was possibly the most beautiful flat in Auckland, with an outdoor upstairs garden. So many lifetimes later I am in Auckland Hospital being treated for prostate cancer. Such a short distance and yet so far ... but it is a great comfort to glance out the window and see an old haunt potent with memory and, in the other direction, the ruffled swan on the gates that led into the Domain, where we had so many picnics as children and later, as a student in various drugged states of either ecstasy or despond, I wandered about thinking I lived in a very beautiful pocket of existence.

November 17, 7.42 a.m.

After the long silence of the night, which begins about 9.15 in Acute Oncology and goes through to the first stirrings round 5.30ish, it's a pleasure to look out the window and see a crisp day with people hurrying off to work. I think of all the times I – likewise – walked past the hospital, screening from my mind all the pain that dwells within, focusing instead on my end objective, or the fact I was running late or early, or when was I going to have a coffee and especially where? It's a tonic for me

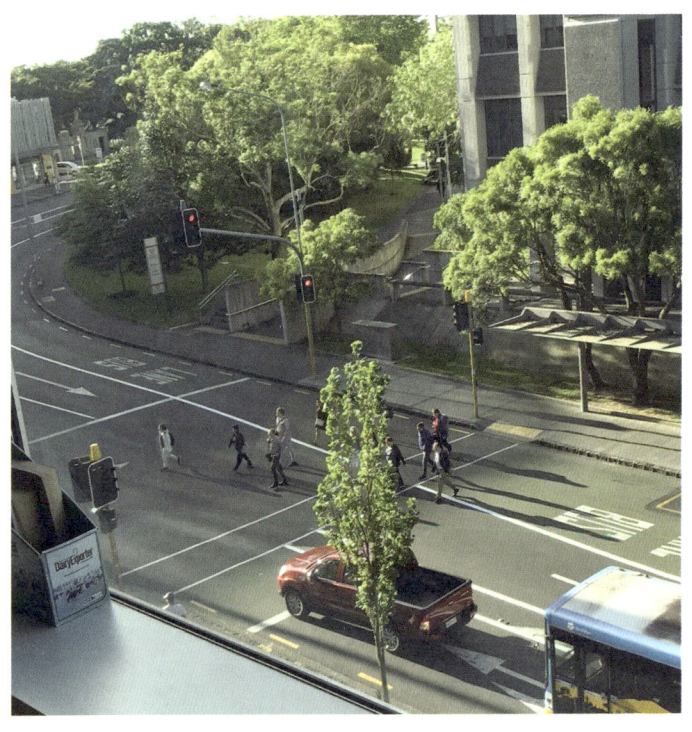

looking out the window now, seeing life going on, everyone out there beautifully engaged in the act of living.

Syntactical correctness: when I asked for 'a pain killer' I was always corrected. It's 'pain relief'. This is because pain cannot be killed. It can only be relieved.

Note to self. It's not a game, you know. It's not a fucking *literary device*.

Later:
It was only today that I realised I was in a ward for men very close to dying. And the strangest fact was I was not an exception. I was one of them.

In praise of Ronnie the nurse:
She has a lived-in face and a voice which speaks of late night music and low lights, a soft husky catch of a voice which always has at its end the suggestion of a laugh. But she's serious, on the level, is Ronnie. 'What's your level of pain, one to ten?' 'Peter, you don't have to be in pain. Right?' 'Right' I mumble, chastened by a lifetime's practice in being stoic. Grateful to give in.

Ronnie sees the joke in things, Ronnie sees what's serious. She's a voice you lilt to the moment she enters the room. It's like a gust of wind filling the space, the energy of an outside world from which we are all momentarily exiled. She carries it in, captures it, and there's some kind of exultation in how she expends it among us. Life force, breath of life.

A professional doing her job, doing the rounds, adding the unseen, unknown but deeply felt.

It is we who are enriched.

Ronnie the nurse: we four men in our separate beds in Room 13A, Ward 64 salute you!

November 19, 9.43 a.m.

Two sides of my life now I'm out of hospital. Grateful, thrilled to be back in 'the land of the living', a little uncertain, loving being home. Friends call and visit, I sleep. Life always has two sides, it's just at the moment I am seeing them clearly now. That isn't necessarily a bad thing. The taste of my first latte was so bound up in anticipation I actually found it hard to analyse what I was feeling/tasting. It's better not to anticipate things maybe – just go with what's happening. For such a controlling person like moi, this is quite some lesson.

Later:
Tomorrow morning I begin the 'radiotherapy' aka radiation which is the first interventionist treatment I have had for the cancer. It terrifies me. I know of the risks – other organs and tissues implicated in the blitz – and I am unhappy giving up my body for something that seems almost grotesquely non-specific.

The fact is I have never had one person sit me down and go through the aetiology of my disease, let alone its prognosis.

Are we merely at a palliative stage – already?

The closest was the urologist telling me over the phone that there was 'quite extensive disease in the bones, the lymph nodes, in the axial skeleton, spine, pelvis and also top of the femur'. (I wrote it down on some paper as he spoke.) It was 'pretty nasty stuff', he said in a cautious, rather quiet voice. There were also minor compression fractures of my lumbar spine. 'Some of the bone has collapsed,' he said. 'There are lesions in the neck of the femur.'

But what does this mean?

A non-communicative and tense radiologist dropped onto my lap a full record of my condition but I lack the specialised knowledge to know how to interpret what it says. But this doesn't sound good: 'There is widespread metastatic disease throughout the spinal column. There is involvement of all vertebrae with abnormal T1 and T2 signal.' So there's metastised cancer in my bones, my back, my spine and in the lymph nodes – the cancer is quite extensive. One side of my back is extensively compromised and may need, says the radiologist coolly, 'a complete hip replacement'.

So it's incurable cancer. I get that. But how fatal and how quick and how slow? How painful? Already I am on extensive morphine, almost hourly doses as well as the slow-release version of the drug (Sevredol).

Is this as good as it gets? I'm terrified all right.

My throat has started hurting, i.e. an infection, which is not a good sign.

Alison, a very old and intimate friend, has offered to become my doctor. Should I ask her to explain the reality of the diagnosis? Or is this something I cannot bring myself to 'understand'?

It's before midnight the night before radiation, and it's time I stopped fretting and 'got some sleep'.

I was aware I was being sharper than I normally was. I had become like someone impatient about time. I am normally too polite, a default of the mock-gentility of my upbringing. (As Douglas is wont to say, 'The Wells family were the only family in Point Chevalier to have footmen.') But now the imperative of drugs, not feeling quite well, uncertainty about even what was happening to me, made me tetchy to the point of rudeness.

But I'm all over the place. When we got home from the first radiography session this morning – I was so frightened I lost all competency to understand the most basic information like 'turn left at the door' – I smelt the soft warm unmown grass and could have cried. I like being at home.

Then I got the very final mock-up of my new book, *Dear Oliver*, on my computer and I was plunged into the future. (The book will come out in May 2018.)

I actually took a paper copy of the cover into hospital with me last week and its familiarity comforted me. (It's me as a nerdy 15-year-old with tears in my eyes on seeing my Napier grandmother. Beside me, Bess, my mother. We're on the tarmac at Whenuapai. It's 1965.)

Suddenly a corridor opens up in front of me and I look into the future (ironically by looking back, at the past).

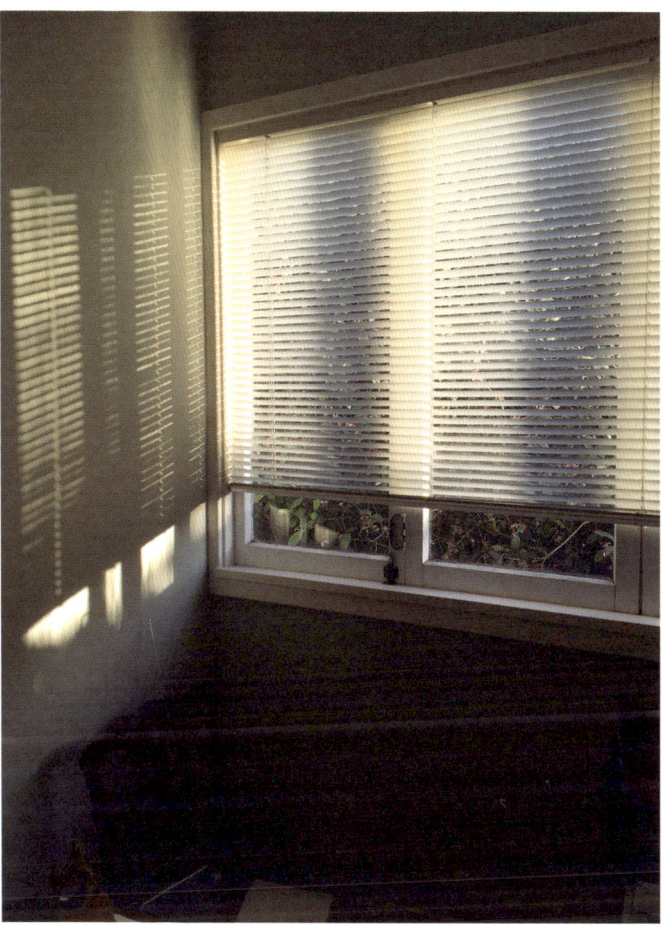

Yet I'm impatient about time at the moment. I have a few other books I want to write, one in rough draft on my desk. So while I am in the trenches of bad temper and uncertainty about my health, not being capable of understanding simple directions like 'turn left' and on the verge of being tetchy and testy . . . I also have a sense of a pale summer sky high and alluring.

November 21, 4.52 a.m.

Ajax the cat stretches out to welcome me home on a stunningly hot Tuesday afternoon. The balm of animals is so appealing. The silence, the empathy, the animal ability to sense sadness, woundedness, and to wordlessly offer companionship.

After radiotherapy I change into pyjamas and lounge about, reading, snoozing, tying up the very last loose threads of *Dear Oliver*. Friends call round, carefully calculating the timing of their visits to around 15 minutes. They bring not only treats – like a child I am very keen on treats – but also the miracle of a friendly face, an empathetic silence and a discreetly watchful gaze. Some say: you must be vigilant and fight. Others say: take your time and recover. Others again say little but share our limited time together and we find ourselves laughing, very agreeably, forgetting for a time the difficult predicament.

Many of these friends I have known over half a lifetime. Some go back to my twenties, some to my thirties and some to my forties. Even they seem very old friends now.

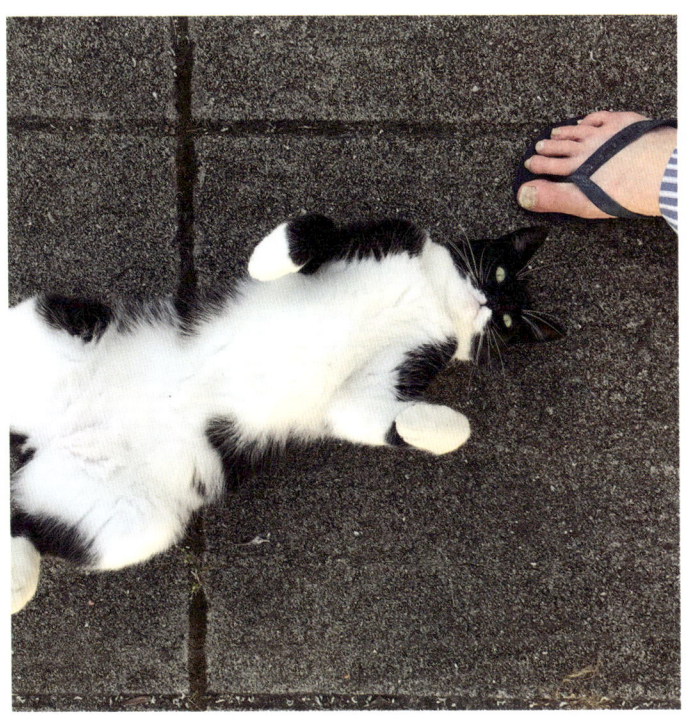

It struck me how these entirely nonsexual relationships have a richness and strength that sexual relationships, which flare up, scorch, immolate, enmadden and flare out, lack. One tends to privilege these sexual relationships. They were what love was *meant* to be like. It ate you alive.

Yet what can one say for the silent depth of friendship based on simpatico natures, a shared sense of humour, respect perhaps for the other's point of view? Knowledge of risks taken, mistakes deeply regretted. Dreams, once vivid, now not so much lost as no longer useful in making one's peace with life. I think of some of the grand erotic madnesses I experienced and confess to finding them, in the light of day, not so very interesting, outside the theatre of self-obsession. I am sustained instead, or perhaps as well as, by the kindly intentions of Ajax the cat as he stretches towards me, turns over and yawns. Or the friends who move towards me to embrace and place their arms carefully about the framework of my ribs but go no further.

November 22, 4.26 a.m.

I had never known pain like that. As a child I had had infected eardrums. That was my definition of the utmost pain a human can stand. Then last night, 10 or so hours after the second dose of radiation, I began to feel a pain so renting I could only cry out, as if in making a sound I was imploring it to stop. It has no dignity and is quite bestial. I'm returning to being an animal in pain.

I can't lie down so am sitting on the side of my bed. I'm afraid to lie down. Especially if the pain suddenly stabs, it becomes impossible not to move without yelling.

Douglas is in another room asleep. We started sleeping separately when my restlessness – my inability to get comfortable – kept him awake. I miss his body enormously, a body that for 26 years has been able to subdue my nervous anxiety, calm me down and make me more human. Even holding hands in the dark is a powerful physical narcotic to me.

I'm afraid to wake him up, but one part of me wants him to be awake, as he could then share my pain. But this is a fact. Nobody can share pain. You can empathise, try to help, calm, obtain medicines, more water, but in the end you are on your own.

Tomorrow (today actually) is Douglas's birthday. I have a small present to give him, then some other presents on the following day when, for practical reasons, we decide to hold a small celebration. Again for practical reasons – I can no longer really manage to cook a meal – we will have Indian takeaways and some Moet. This is not how we expected it to be. But this is how it has turned out.

It's quiet now – as much as Auckland is ever quiet. Cars on the motorway, for example, the restless sounds of people going about their lives. I pray for sleep, for a dulling of pain. I will email the radiologist tomorrow and ask her if I need further pain relief. Really I am asking: is this right?

Later:
I spend the night sitting upright on a dining chair. Somehow this makes me feel like someone from a nineteenth century Russian novel, I'm not sure why. At 8 a.m. I ring the nurses

who specialise in responses to radiation. The woman is mid-conversation when she lifts the phone, is practical, pragmatic, and has seen it all before. I feel an outbreak of relief. We arrange for Douglas and me to come in an hour early, bringing all my meds. She will put me in touch with Hospice Services who specialise in managing pain. She makes me feel as if all this were infinitely possible. As Ronnie said, 'You know, Peter, you don't have to feel pain.'

But more than this, it ends my experience of the overwhelming isolation of extreme pain. So I'm not on my own. And in the meantime, since I still cannot lie down flat without going into convulsions, I will go back to snoozing upright on my Russian dining-room chair . . .

Later:

I am re-admitted to Ward 64. The admitting nurse turns to Douglas and, with reference to me, says, 'You're what? His son?' For some reason this cheers me up and makes me think of when we were new to one another and Douglas had suddenly been admitted to hospital for a small but urgent operation. When he was going under, the nurse said to him, 'Don't worry. When you wake up, your father will be sitting there.' 'I fucking hope not!' was Douglas's spirited rejoinder, and the nurse later admitted, red faced, she was incredibly embarrassed. This made me laugh and laugh at the time – I was glad we were not an identikit gay couple mirroring one another – and sitting here now, awaiting a bed upstairs in Ward 64, intensely relieved my pain will be looked after, it still has the ability to make me smile. We match with whoever we match.

To my utter amazement and like something from a fairy tale, a lithe elderly lady on a walking stick walked into my room smiling and hand delivered a gift from Lyn Kriegel, a Facebook friend. She had come from Karekare. I asked her to sit down and apologised for not being able to make her a cup of tea. She explained it was no trouble. She had caught a train into town, then had a dentist appointment (the numbness was wearing off). She had walked over Grafton Bridge, then managed to find me in this labyrinth (amazing, since I was shifted only an hour ago).

Her face shone with kindness and a kind of grace only intelligent old age can emanate. We chatted about Auckland, Lone Kauri Road, and then she leapt to her feet saying it was time she moved on and was gone.

I shook her hand before she went, partly to convince myself she was real. A visit from a goode faery, I felt.

'What do we live for but to make life a little less difficult for each other' – George Eliot

The radiology specialist said to me it was possible the extreme pain I experienced two nights ago – three? – is actually an expression of how effective the radiation is at killing the cancer. I'd like to think so and I guess we shall see.

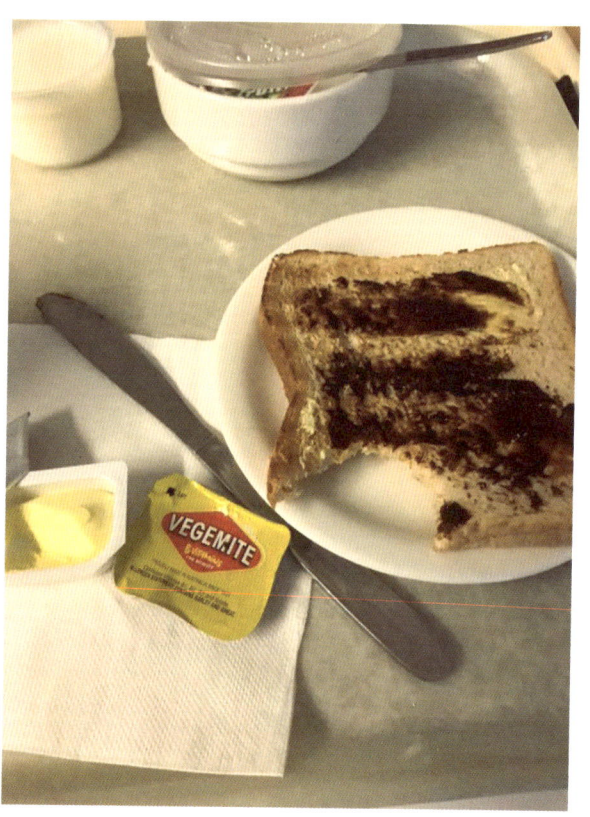

10.04 a.m.

The remarkable taste experiment by which an inevitably cold, thin piece of bread that was once 'toasted' has been left to rest so it takes on a true cardboard consistency. It is then delivered to your room on a stone cold plate, alongside oleaginous matter of a yellowy substance and a more substantial, nay even desperate, dark noxious mixture known as Vegemite. And in your desperation and boredom and hunger you smear said contents across dry cardboard, open your mouth, take a bite and receive the information that there is no pity in existence, only hospital breakfasts. Nevertheless you resolve to 'look on the bright side of life', telling yourself it will only take a moment. You persevere and you eat every last crumb. 'Delicious!' you mentally instruct yourself, while your tastebuds cower and plead never to be so discriminated against again. The sad tale of the Vegemite toast here endeth.

November 25, 4.11 a.m.

At times I open my eyes and I'm surprised to find I'm in a hospital room. I look around me and adjust. It's by no means painful or awkward now – it's just a new kind of normal – and I ask myself, 'How did I end up here?'

It takes me a while for my mind to travel back, branching off at emergency stops, sudden moments of fright, meetings at which these fears seem addressed, only to find later that one small detail unaddressed turned out to be the one significant thing that would pull you back into hospital.

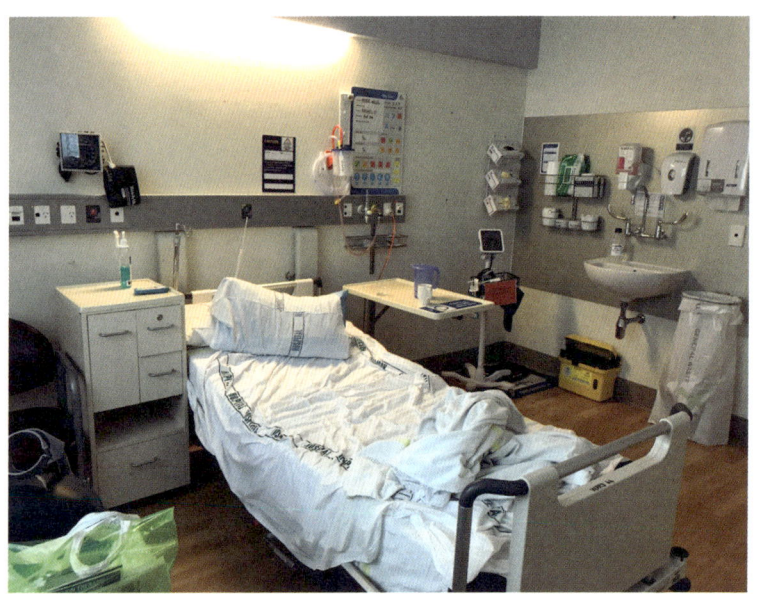

Yet once you're in here it's such a self-sufficient, self-perpetuating system, it's very tempting to give in. (The pain killers help.) It seems to function without you, yet you seem part of its function. Endless pleasant people appear to ask questions, often the same questions over again.

Occasionally you must disturb yourself, so you struggle in your hazy mind to connect the pertinent facts so that the one unaddressed small problem does not open up before your feet again. (Hospice Pain Management seems so ideal but you have no reference point or address, for example.)

You are either close to dying or you are infinitely distant. You are intimate now with the idea – but only the idea – of death, and you are not sure you want to get any closer. Isn't a vague impression kinder at times? Besides, who can read the sentence? 'I'm an eleven-year survivor of cancer,' an acquaintance said to me the other day. There are no rules. Take medicinal dope. Take turmeric. Just try and remember all the pills and what they're meant to be doing to you and for you.

Be grateful. Be grateful you're alive and we have a hospital system which still functions. Just be grateful.

And lie back on that bed in Ward 64 Room 5 thinking of all the stories you've heard, so spliced open in the urgency and heartbreak of the moment. Feel humble to be so near the human condition.

The pain killer eases your blood through your veins. You wonder if you're not being sentimental. You wonder if you don't actually like being removed from life and wrapped up in cotton wool and protected.

Then you hear the rattle of a wheelchair coming closer. The orderly has arrived to wheel you down to 'Transition'.

Transition is where you're headed. The cotton wool is taken away. The plugs taken out of your arms. You say – momentarily, like a schoolboy leaving a boarding school he suspects he'll never escape – the cheerful goodbyes of strangers who hope never to see one another again, at the same time accepting that when you do meet again, inevitably, you will be familiar and hail-fellow well-met.

Then at the last moment that young doctor with a smooth face unfurrowed by life's harsh teachings – the one who gave you marching orders this morning – pops back in. 'By the way, have you got enough Sevredol to get on with at home?' No Blanche du Bois could have answered with a deeper curtsey.

This is a new kind of transition for me. In *Dear Oliver* I talk about how aging is as much a philosophical experience as a bodily one. Being sick, ill or whatever it's called – experiencing cancer – is the same. It's not only an illness, an attack, but it's a kind of new learning, with all its ability to not connect, to lose meaning or project new translucencies. I'm trying to listen, to hear, to negotiate what is patently a difficult and complex course. But it is also an education in the human emotions, not least my own.

3.54 p.m.
Why I am happy to be home . . . in the time I was in hospital it has magically turned to summer.

November 26, 4.54 a.m.

Feeling my way down the back steps by touch – I was going out to turn a hose off – the most delicious apprehension of an early summer night, air alive with insects and sounds and a drowsy wind barely stirring: I felt I was walking out into a primeval memory of summer evenings I knew as a child. I am no longer a child but in that second I felt all the longing and anticipation of another summer.

3.39 p.m.

This morning I felt energised so got up early. The dishes from last night's meal were there. I had slow-roasted a small leg of lamb – as much for the smell as the taste. (I'll make a shepherd's pie in a day, my all-time favourite comfort food.) We had drunk some good champagne.

I've been reading Atul Gawande's *Being Mortal: Illness, Medicine and What Matters in the End*. Partly this is because I'm seeing a consulting oncologist tomorrow and I have little idea what to ask.

Reading the book is not without its challenges. For example: 'A study led by the sociologist Nicholas Christakis asked the doctors of almost 500 terminally ill patients to estimate how long their patient would survive, then followed the patients. 63% of doctors overestimated their patient's survival time. Just 17% underestimated it.'

Gawande's thing is that people suffering terminal conditions need to be more assertive about how much they want to do to try to change what may be, at some time or another, a predestined end. '. . . those who saw a palliative care specialist stopped chemotherapy sooner, entered hospice far earlier, experienced less suffering at the end of their lives – and they lived 25 per cent longer.'

This is all a lot for me to think about. I have even to work out where I lie within this perspective. I do not know at present. There has been a lot of 'It's not good but it's not the worst I've seen.'

I was taken aback on the day I left hospital, on Friday, when that smooth-faced young doctor mentioned to me the likelihood I would be having chemotherapy. This was a shock. I had understood it was a distant possibility. Now I saw the doors were wide open and they were in fact awaiting me. It was I who had to catch up.

So on this gentle Sunday I see friends, we laugh, I do a bit of writing, read some more Gawande then decide I can't bear to read any more. I have a Sunday snooze and I plan to have a piece of that delicious date loaf Alexa brought round. It was warm from the oven when she arrived.

Also I have a washing basket of mismatched socks to match up. This suddenly seems rather enjoyable.

Concentrate on the actual, I think.

November 28, 2.33 a.m.

The empathy of cats. Of animals. At my worst, when my Napier doctor said I had prostate cancer and it was too late to do anything – 'Here's some Paracetamol and goodbye' – I was in hell. Douglas was up in Auckland and I wanted to talk to him face to face. It was a long and terrible night. But the two

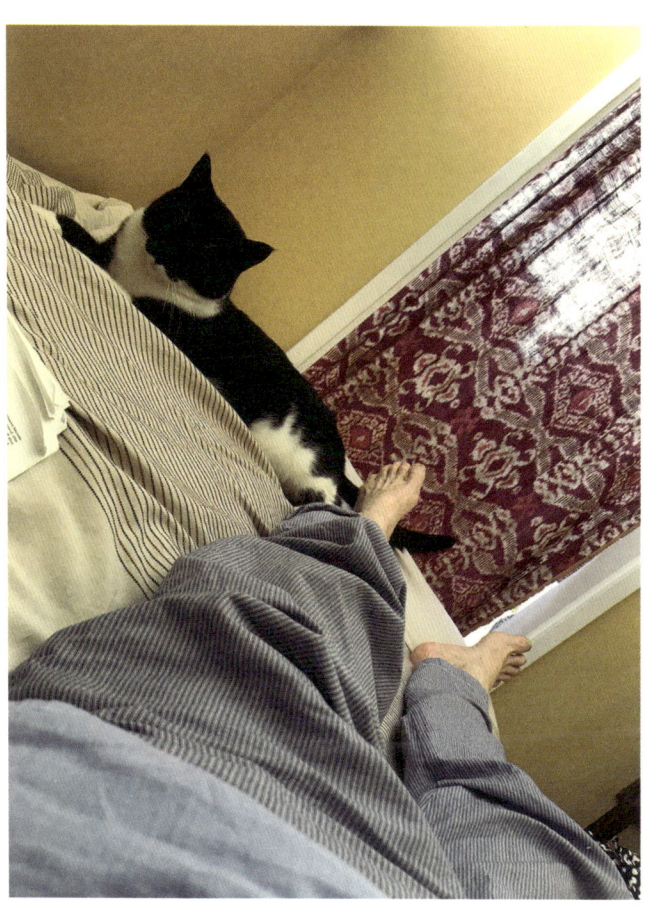

cats we have in Napier came and slept close to the edge of my bed. There was a real delicacy in that they did not impinge on my territory, so, as I was thrashing to and fro, they were not in the way. They stayed close by my bed all night, sentinels.

This arvo, feeling a little fragile from my morning's zap of radiography, Ajax the cat very quietly jumped up on the bed, placed himself near my feet, not touching me, looked at me intensely for a long moment, then went to sleep. It touched me deeply.

I'm juggling in my mind the realities of accepting an 18-week course of chemo after Christmas. I've decided to try an early 'aggressive' response, though some wan dubious part of me wonders if it is to myself, rather than the cancer, that the aggression happens. Or are we the same? An interesting question.

I have a lot of questions in my mind at the moment. (Costs, pain, loss of sex, danger. Will it even work?)

The good thing is I am through 'the immediate crisis' that exploded in mid-October. Now I am in the 'treatment phase'. I have doctors here in Auckland taking able and astute care of me. I feel I can plan my life ahead. Surely this is a corner? And isn't it good symbolism that, after visiting the oncologist and deciding to go ahead with a plan of treatment, the very final tweaks of *Dear Oliver* were done, so now my new book can wing its way into the future. I am listening to the beat of its wings as I sleep . . .

November 29, 3.17 a.m.

If someone had said to me two months ago 'You can only walk with crutches', I would have looked at them with disbelief. Yet walking on crutches has crept up on me and I have got, if not fond of them, to regard the sight of them as a relief. They hold me up while I drag my sorry arse around God's earth.

I'm still trying to work out a way round the problem when people say, 'Hey what happened?' 'Problems with my back' seems close enough to the truth without going into detail. Whose business is it anyway?

Disclosure is a strange thing. I've chosen Facebook as my way of talking about what's happening to me, which is curious as it's so porous yet, I've found, so listening. I have had my moments of self-pity, especially at the start, but somehow I've travelled speedily into acceptance. Perhaps dear old Bess, my mother, dying in April did not harden me but prepared me for life's precariousness. (I still wish I could look into her face.)

November 30, 5.23 a.m.

Probably the most alone I've been on this 'journey' (don't know what to call it at the moment) is when I've been going through scans or having radiography/radiation. It's a really weird experience, as it's here, for the first time, you're presented with the information that you/your body and your 'disease' (right term?) are one and the same and you need to present/submit your body for impartial, scientific investigation or attempted remedy.

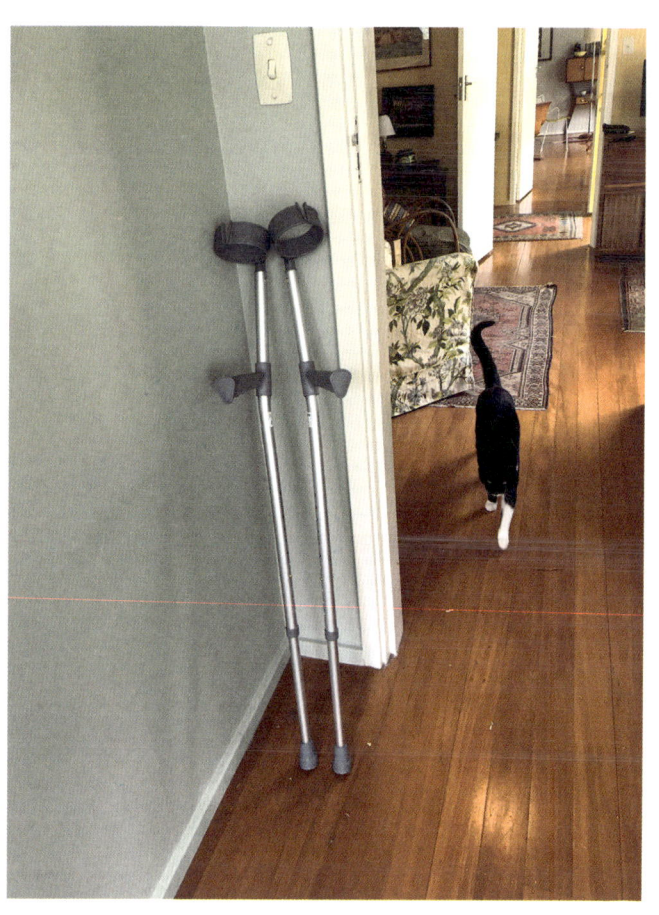

You are inevitably lying down on a relatively narrow plank-like support. Comfort will be minimal as it's important nothing intervenes between your flesh and 'the machine'. Sometimes you cross your arms on your chest like a medieval saint, and you are always asked to stay as still as possible.

None of these procedures takes long in objective time, but those five or ten minutes of utter isolation, in a room rendered so dangerous that all other living beings evacuate, has a way of extending time into a philosophical inquiry: how did I end up here? How did this happen?

Pondering this takes up a certain amount of time. Then you begin to wonder how much more time there is to go. Big question: eyes open or eyes shut.

In the claustrophobic tunnel of an MRI scan I keep my eyes closed in the hope I will evade panic. They play radio music, sometimes asking what station you'd like. (When I said RNZ, this seemed unusual.) Once it was rap music and I sort of lay there and sighed.

Radiation tends to have strange effects after eight or so hours, but at the time it is eerily effectless. It doesn't even hurt. Yesterday, celebrating the fact it was my last zap, I lay there with my eyes open, watching the strangely dull grey machine parts changing their format around me. There are pauses, buzzes, nothing particularly stressful. A red light goes on. It's just like you're a mouse inside a machine. And that machine is something from an old 1950s sci-fi film, never quite believable.

But you have been reminded of your subjectness earlier when they prepared your body for the zap. Here you have to be as passive as possible and they push and prod you into the refinement of the best possible position. This is utterly key so all you can do is lie there – and give up.

It's somewhere between this strange, reluctant compliance and a sturdier inner voice that I reside. Yesterday I watched the dance of the radiation machine; I looked at the projected image of trees in blossom on the tiled ceiling, working out it was America; noted the hanging mike into which I could theoretically have spoken. Then somehow abruptly I fell asleep and it was only when I felt fingers on my stomach that I realised it was over and that a bright and cheerful staff member was chatting to me, hurrying me on my way while I lay on my back trying to work out how to pull my pants back up over my nakedness and then somehow manage to revolve upright without causing too much pain. She then began spraying where I lay with, I guess, some disinfectant as a form of farewell.

'Hope we don't see you again!' we say as I hobble away. I meet D outside and we rush off to have an early morning coffee in a cafe where I celebrate being out in the living world and everything appears both very precious and beautifully normal.

Later:
My mind lingers, caught on a skein of words in a report sent from the oncologist to the urologist. Under the heading 'Social History' it says: '. . . we have been through the diagnosis of metastatic prostate cancer. He had already understood that this was not curable and we have discussed how the anti-androgen therapy and the hormone LHRH agonist function . . . We have also discussed the role of chemotherapy in early use and hormone sensitive prostate cancer and the possible around 18 months benefit from this over and above the many years of life most patients would have from use of the standard hormone therapy.'

What does this mean?

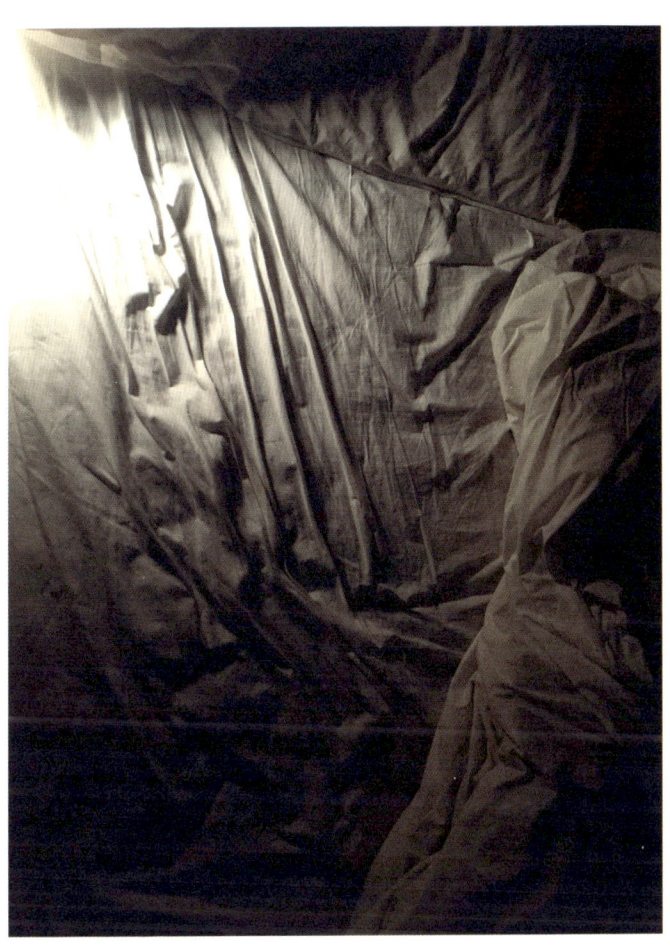

My mind seems on a strange level at the moment, barely functional. Or rather, I am looking beneath or hearing under or seeing other things. Most of all I need to sleep. But what does this mean?

'Not curable' I understand. 'Possible around 18 months benefit . . . Over and above the many years of life most patients would have from use of the standard hormone therapy . . .'? Am I getting an extra 18 months?

I feel intense relief when D comes to interviews with me, as he remembers dates, times, when and where. I'm almost inert in these interviews, struggling to make sense of what is obvious and logical as well as what is quite difficult to grasp.

This strange listening silence I hear is not unpleasant though, and swells at night (and hence why I often post in the very early hours of the morning: this is when I feel most at home).

December 1, 2.27 a.m.

Old friends as bookends.

Today two old friends arrived round with lunch. I met Jenny when she was just over 17 and Alexa when she was 16. I was 20, gay and a student. I am 67 now and our bond is such they wander in the door, put down a gorgeous lunch and conversation never stops. It is like a big bolt of cloth unrolling from our long-ago youth and rolling off into the future with the same energy, humour, insight and – generosity.

As I open the door to greet them, it's as if a light floods in – as it did this evening through the plane window as I flew with D back to Napier.

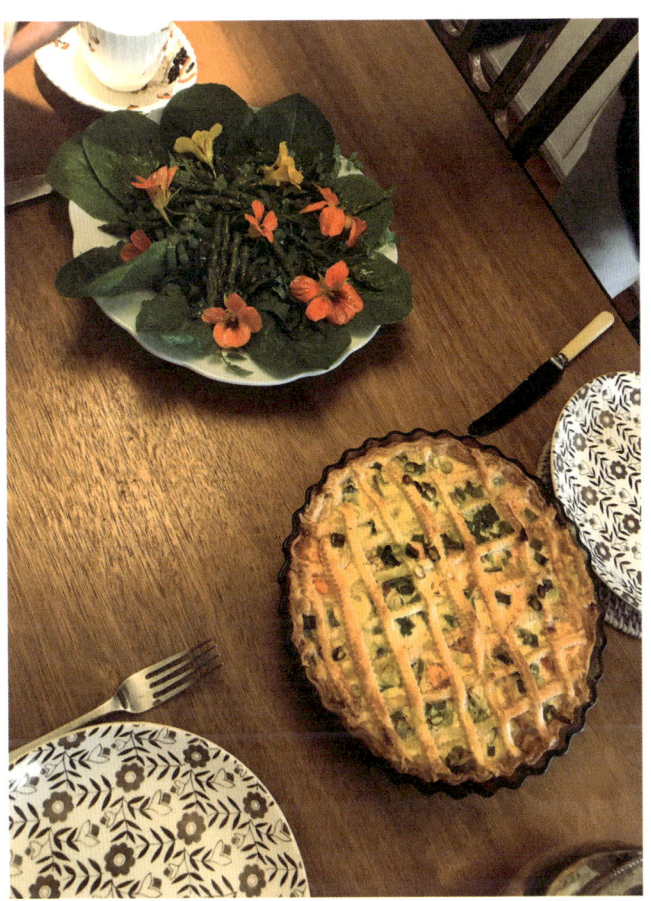

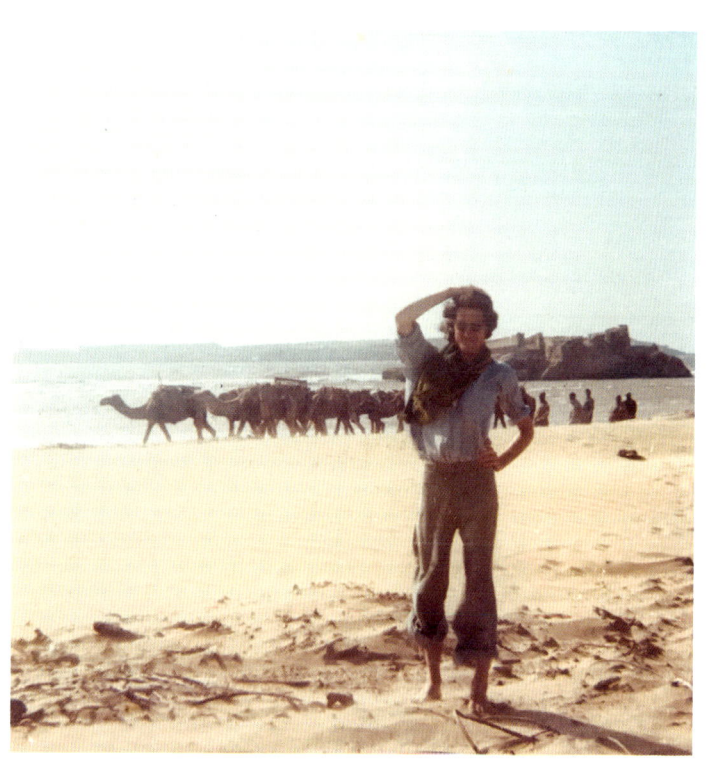

December 2, 12 a.m.

Taking a break. Going through old photos. Writing names on the back: *Me at 25. Outside Essaouira, Morocco, 1975.* I'm getting beautifully lost, as you can only at 25, in a foreign country, when there seems so much time . . .

I got the idea for the first story I would ever get published on this holiday, so it also marks a beginning.

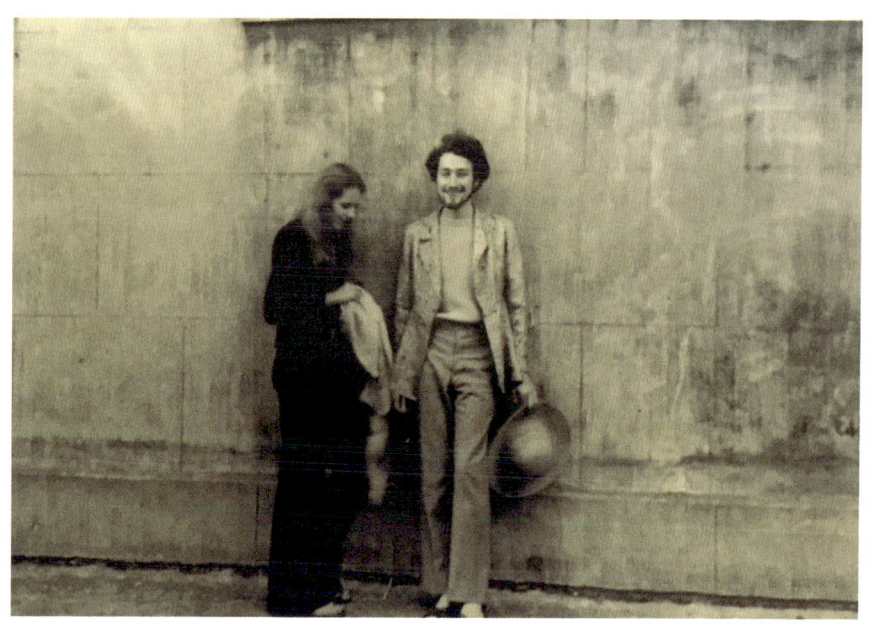

Taking a break, part 2. The other day I posted about old friends Alexa and Jenny bringing me lunch. This is a photo from when Jenny Maidment and I were flatmates in the early '70s. The photo captures us on our way home from the Hot House at the Winter Gardens. Inevitably we had had a smoke to enjoy its beauty.

We were very simpatico, great friends, and shared a ludicrous sense of humour which I think this photo captures. We were in love with Bertolucci and Visconti films. My jacket was pale-blue Chinese silk and I had a large Bloomsbury-style straw hat but I see I am wearing Roman sandals. Jenny was naturally elegant and was great at mimicking people. I wish I could remember what she had just said that made me so happy.

Little did we think over 40 years later we would still share a sense of humour, outrage over politics, and the simpler elemental thing of a bridge of memories over which we crossed to find ourselves in this complex present.

To friends, wherever they be.

7.47 p.m.

This (page 36) is a photo of me from the late 1970s, probably taken in Northland. I had come back to Muldoon's NZ at a time of record outward migration – the period of 'the last person to leave, turn out the lights'. I went against the tide and, after writing and studying in the UK, I made an emotional commitment to come back and invest whatever talents, energy and vision I had in what was here. It was like a promise I made.

I was a very serious young man, committed and earnest; I was also in love with this difficult place, which as Allen

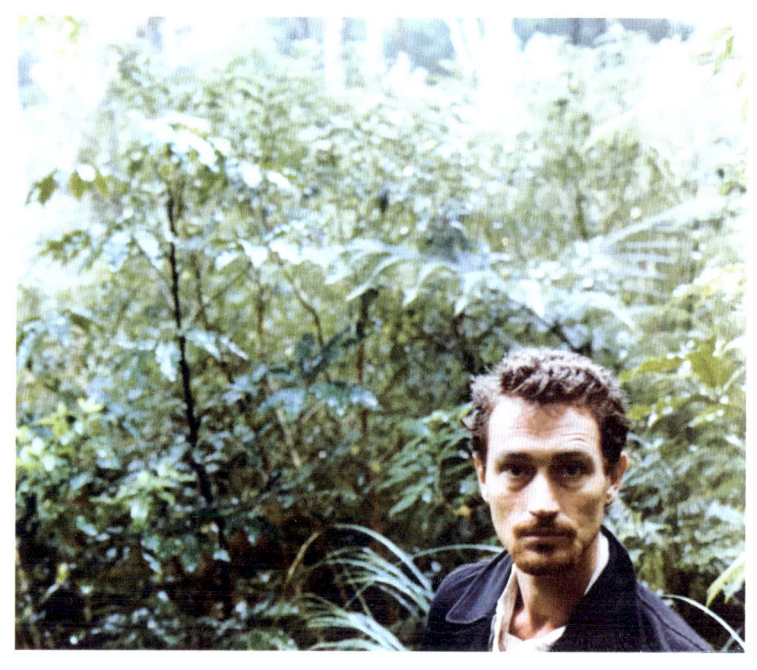

Curnow has said, is 'under described'. Maybe that is all in my look – love, searching, actually the act of looking itself.

There's something in the intensity of the look – the way I am placed so strangely within the landscape. It takes me back to all those hopes and dreams.

I had a young man's face just as it was maturing into the face I would carry into the future, to settle into age itself. As for that thick auburn hair . . . where did it go?

December 5, 2.49 a.m.

Then there was the time I got into trouble. Terrible trouble. I was too earnest and too angry. This photo (page 38) was taken the day after the scandal sheet *Truth* revealed to an outraged public that I was what they termed 'The GOFTA Slob'.

At the time of this photo I thought the whole thing was a bit of a joke. It was even a notch on my belt to have become, as the sub-headline said, 'The Man Who Shocked the Nation'.

Hence the smirk. (And mullet.)

Not so. Backtrack. On the night of the 1987 Film and Television Awards I had yelled out 'Fuck off, sexist shit' to John Inman of *Are You Being Served?* when he came on the stage. Context: it was 1987 and we were fighting for homosexual rights, and Inman represented a character who could never be authentically gay, i.e. he could never say who he was. A strange person to give out an award in such contentious times.

Further context: I had co-written and then directed a 30-minute drama called *Jewel's Darl* which, in the context of

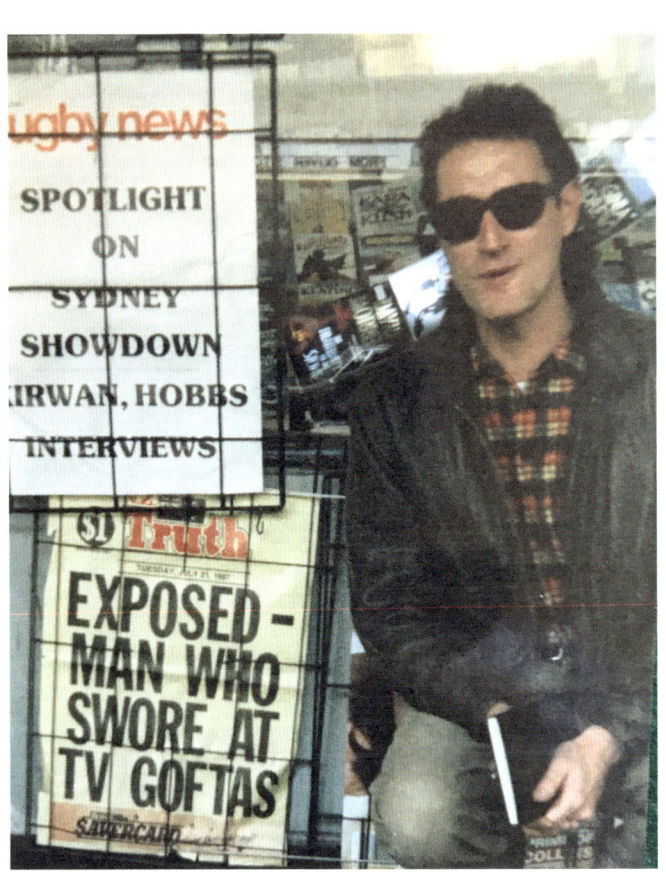

the sexual politics of the period, was radical and out there. It was about a day in the life of a transgender woman and her transvestite friend. TVNZ had objected to trans people being treated as anything other than 'Benny Hill' funny and had sat on it for a year. When Inman came onstage I'd just missed out on a prize for best directing, best writing, and then best film. I was feeling pretty raw.

Further context: I had no idea the awards were being broadcast live, with no delay. Fuck was not a word commonly heard on public television in those days. It was a very big deal.

The following weeks and months revealed the depth of my offence.

My career was on the point of blossoming. I was making a documentary aimed at saving Auckland's Civic Theatre from demolition. Ahead lay a mini-feature about de-stigmatising AIDS at the time when AIDS hysteria ruled the world. Even a feature film (*Desperate Remedies*) lay ahead in the dim future.

I got anonymous phone calls: *Get AIDS and die, homo.* People no longer met my eye. 'Friends' melted away. I became a non-person in the industry, my career pushed to the side, starved of funds for future projects. I became persona non grata and a laughing stock.

So it did turn out to be a big deal. For years afterward I knew people much preferred to remember me – pigeonhole me – as the Gofta Slob, rather than the person who helped save the Civic Theatre or, later, helped create the Auckland Writers Festival.

It's a reflection on human nature that people often prefer to belittle than to celebrate.

Over time I got over it. But did my love affair with NZ – that thing which brought me back to NZ with such a desire to contribute – did that survive? It was seriously dented. At that moment I felt I'd looked right into the heart of a cold, miserablist country.

The GOFTA period marks a time as narrow as a bridge: on one side, the part of my life 'before GOFTA'; on the other, life after it. In time I would leave the film and television industry. I turned more to writing, as the page seemed safer – I could be more in control.

But it did give me some life skills.

Steel entered my soul. When people comment now that I am managing to look at my current difficulties with at least some equanimity – some acceptance – it is because I learnt survival skills at that time.

As a footnote I'd add that when John Inman died, many young gay men reflected that it was people like him who made them terrified to come out. 'If that's what I've got to be like, I'd rather stay in.' So role models and fair representation do matter.

It's a long time ago and I understand better now that Inman's winking, leering comedy related to illegality and persecution – to what you could never say out loud. But I still shudder at my naivety in thinking that calling him out was 'all a bit of a joke' and it would be over in the next news cycle. It changed my life.

In fact, it has taken me a painful 30 years to write anything about it – which is what this post is here.

Later:
The Salon des Refuses was where artists who were refused the right to appear in more established art spaces decided to hold their own defiant exhibitions. After I was disgraced by

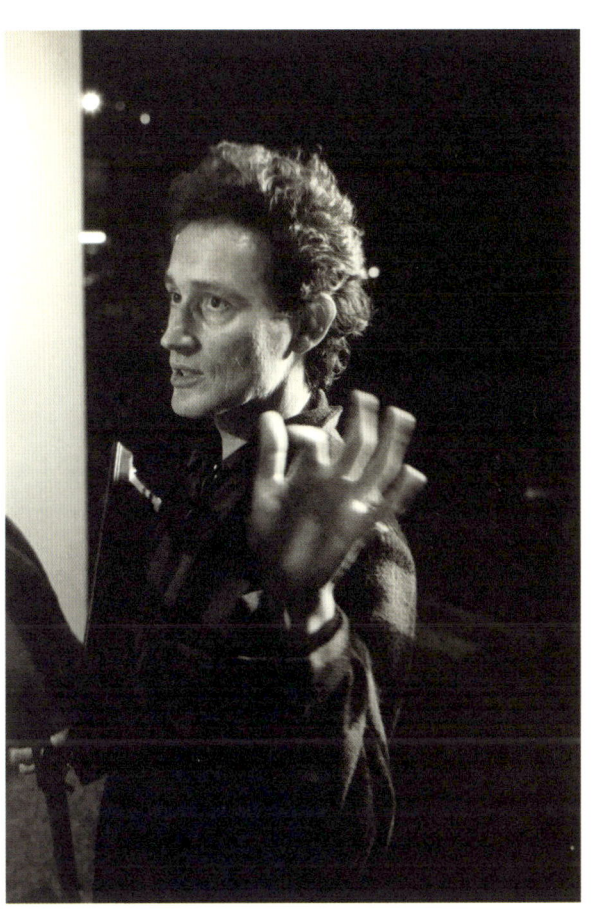

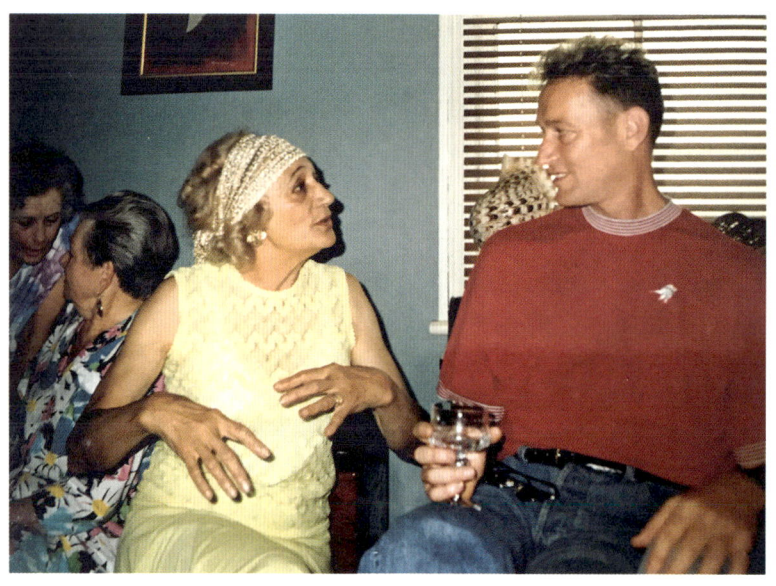

the GOFTA incident I found myself unexpectedly popular at a most extraordinary gathering. This was held at the home of Diana Wong, a Chinese New Zealand-born film-maker from the 1970s. She lived in Grey Lynn in the house she was born in. Her parents were market gardeners who had a very successful shop at the bottom of Queen Street when shops and even a cinema flowed right down to the Ferry Buildings. Diana invited me to an afternoon tea. Here there was a group of people I had never met before – apart from Freda Stark, the scandaleuse of the Mighty Civic Theatre. It was all very jolly.

Gradually, over the years, I began to understand it was a form of salon des refuses – it was a gathering of people who didn't fit in the remorselessly conformist society of the 1950s and 1960s (like Diana herself, a highly articulate forthright Chinese woman).

The soirées included a woman who was Auckland's first woman taxi driver (exceptionally brave in the loutish 1960s); a well-known woman ventriloquist – there was always a sprinkle of red velvet and magic in the air; Freda, the survivor of a 1937 murder trial and lesbian scandal; her nephew, the highly camp pianist and conversationalist Billie Farnell.

People would play the pianola: an old '40s or '50s movie might be playing. A woman who was a window dresser at Smith & Caughey's talked to the formidable Ramai Hayward, the Māori wife of the legendary film-maker Rudall, an actor and a film-maker (I think) in her own right.

So this is a very much younger me listening to 'Dame' Ramai, as I always called her in my mind. She is in full flight. In the background, stage left, you can just see the 'mannish hairstyle' of Freda Stark who is in full gossip mode with a woman magician. I no longer bear the wounds of the GOFTA fiasco. I had fallen in love. Just at the very corner of the shot you can see my hand resting on the knee of Douglas, whom I had met relatively recently. We were in that stage of being in love when you can't bear to be physically apart for more than a second. Nauseating for everyone else, it's a kind of magical period for those happily occupying the house of love.

So this is the other side of the coin of the GOFTA fiasco. I was welcomed into a coven of highly unusual people, all of whom, at some point, had fallen foul of the conformist times – yet in that noisy room, full of opinion and brio, I knew I was in a very special and even honorific space. I was welcomed in.

December 6, 3.03 a.m.

Yesterday, on the spur of the moment, I decided there was no reason I could not jettison my crutches and have a go at driving the car. I was in Napier where traffic is relatively light. I chucked the crutches in the back, perhaps a touch brutally; got in the driver's seat and backed down the drive. Nothing happened. Or rather my limbs obeyed a lifetime's devotion to and pleasure in driving. With what eerie ease I flew down the hill to the supermarket where I parked the car, got my crutches out, did the shopping, then – in a blaze of triumph – took the shopping home.

I was reminded of the first steep downward hill when I got a push bike – a compound of exhilaration, disbelief and utter pleasure in being alive.

Then today in Auckland I got in the mail a 'disability parking pass'. Instead of feeling this was part of my downward trend towards immobility, I noted it went through to 'November 2022'. In a world in which no one will or can give me dates, this struck me as wondrous. It seemed full of confidence, ebullience, and mentally I stuck it before me, like a badge I could flash at people as I 'drove into the future', waving almost like a beauty queen.

Later:
Occasionally when I look at FB more closely, perhaps analytically, I lose my nerve. Aren't my postings completely unlike all the others to the point they make me a freak? I have been mainlining a form of truth – there is no point in deception or vanity.

I had only my iPhone when I first ended up in Acute Oncology and a small space within the screen on which to register my own truth or my own sense of disarray. I have begun to worry lately, however, that I have been presenting a person who has somehow come to terms with a limited life duration in an unreal way. The fact is my mood drifts all the time. I sleep a lot. I don't necessarily find information easy to integrate mainly because my mind is all over the place. I have moments of terrible pain followed by anxiety. And I realise I have started to use FB postings just to trace where my errant mind will go.

Hence the issue of GOFTA suddenly emerging. I was able to somehow contextualise it in a way I had never been able to before. I 'understood' it and no longer sublimated all the grief and pain I felt at the time – the shame I had brought on the family name and myself.

Not being able to stand the bullshit any longer is one way to put it.

I decided in the flush of the situation to let it go ahead. I would 'publish' or post whenever and whatever I wanted: in such a restrictive situation as an incurable illness this felt very freeing. 'Is it any good?' 'Where is it going?' These are questions I occasionally ask myself. I don't know. All I know is I keep having ideas and these ideas are helping me stay alive. (As well as the echoes that keep coming back from FB friends . . . that too, definitely.)

Later again:
Steve Braunias got in touch asking if The Spinoff could post these meanderings. I said yes, then was attacked by fear. Would it be the same? Would I become self-conscious, arch? Christ. Or can I keep dawdling along the grass strip by the main road. I don't want to 'think about what I write'.

David Herkt, a seasoned friend, says I need to be 'aware of PR and their magnifications'. This frightens me, as intimacy is all I've got. All. 'People will be intimate with your health.' 'You will have to deal with unsolicited consequences.' This is why you have friends. To warn you. To see what's behind you. To see what you can't see. Then he adds a brilliant rejoinder which cheers me up. 'I've grown up in public with my pants down. I was simply being explicit about consequences. God knows I have, like you, laid it all on the line often enough. I think people need to be relentlessly honest or else how are we going to learn, huh?'

Within seconds an imessage appears: Hi. How you doing today handsome

December 7, 3.09 a.m.

Having posted tonight's meanderings on FB, then for the first time sent them off to Steve Braunias at The Spinoff, I go back to bed and instead of easing back into sleep I lie there worriting. How will this new and public outing change what I'm writing – especially when it has no theme or overall objective apart from registering what's happening. Almost so I can understand it myself?

Will people – 'people' – have opinions and want to express them? Worse, 'reach out' when my body is this maggot-hung cave which shrieks with warning klaxons at the thought of being touched. Who is fooling who? Will I have to dress up to open the door? Who am I fooling? When I said 'intimacy is all I've got. All.' – that was not rhetoric.

Or do I just carry on as if 'nothing has changed'? Well, what has changed? As my father would say, 'You've started making a fool of yourself in public.' Or my mother: 'People don't want to know that. Have you no modesty? No shame.'

Shame, my old companion, my old prison guard, my old familiar. I lost shame somewhere along the way. I lost it when I became a writer or, more to the point, a diary or journal keeper.

But that isn't what's keeping me awake. There's a slight twinge on my left side back – the side I'm lying on. I've taken two Sevredol which the nurse from the hospice assured me is morphine but in a light dosage. I try and imagine the future – not only of my body but also the body of my writing. I can't see how it's going to go and I realise this worriting is just my way of trying to calm myself down.

The night train judders by reassuringly. The night-time sounds strike me as familiar, almost kind. It is not cold now at

47

dawn and I'm not really in pain. I have books beside me lined up to read.

(When SB asked me for a title I chose impulsively 'Hello Darkness'. The alternative was that slightly intrusive, 'Peter, what's on your mind?' that appears every time I open FB. I guess 'Hello Darkness' is seen as a sentimental choice. Maybe I have to just remember that sense of intimacy – talking in and to the dark. For the fact is I am an almost morbidly private person. But talking in the dark – talking to the dark – posting at 3.09 a.m. seems to me familiar, ordinary and more to the point necessary. Go figure.)

December 8, 4.12 a.m.

You start out the night thinking it's going to be okay. You have a bath maybe, you're relaxed. Besides there's still acres of A.N. Wilson on Tolstoy to go and you're feeling frankly tired. You won't take Sevredol tonight. You laze around and it's true you do drift off, but disappointingly your watch shows it's just past midnight and suddenly you get this sense of the expanse of the night. But you're cool about it – after all you've been doing it for a while now. You get out your phone, check if there are any new messages. You read a little and suddenly the book is tilting over in your hand and you succumb to sleep.

It's past three now and it's very quiet. It's not unpleasant – you just wish you could sleep. Maybe a Sevredol wouldn't be such a bad idea. You take one, counting them carefully, remembering the hospice nurse saying they were really quite low in morphine. But since when did you start measuring your morphine intake? It's part of your changed condition. You just accept it. You go to sleep, sort of. Time for a toilet stop. Is it number ones or the more humiliating number twos? You're not quite in control of things here now – something that would have once horrified you. Now you don't so much not accept it as see it as part of the landscape of the medication you're on. It's all start stop open shut. Handle it.

You're back in your room. Time to check out the New York Times app. You love the NYT app. You can row into the deep silence of the night, going from books to movies to theatre – you can check out wedding styles, diets, obituaries – but you feel slightly depressed when you read Harvey Weinstein needed injections to get erect so he could then go round freaking out all those women. You think of the tragedy of the human condition – it seems suddenly bleak. It's very quiet now.

Not a bad time to get on to Tolstoy, who has now written the first draft of *Anna Karenina* in three weeks, before he goes back and changes Anna from a misshapen ugly woman to the febrile creature we all know and love. Now it gets interesting. Wilson says Tolstoy limbers up reading English novels. He's a great fan of Trollope. This quietly thrills me, and Wilson asserts the English novel in Anna's hand on the train is actually Trollope's *The Prime Minister*. This thrills me again. Life seems suddenly coherent.

I get up and do a post on Facebook, turning the light on and closing my study door. This also makes my life seem coherent. Have a meaning. But it's still only 4.12 a.m., is it too early to go and have a cup of tea? My crutch is noisy, I have to be careful. I go and look in D's room. He's beautifully chaotically asleep, Ajax sprawled out like an all-conquering wolf pressed to his side. It's two hours before I can make D his morning coffee and bring it to him, a ritual I enjoy even though these days I have to manage crutch and steaming latte bowl and not spill it as I hobble along.

'This poor old cripple', I called myself to D this evening, smiling. He laughed too. It seems like a joke even though within it is a frightening possibility. But we still smile and laugh and I long for his touch even though the framework of my body feels, as I said to a young friend, as if it's hung with jagged crystal maggots (laughing here).

You have to be a little sardonic. To survive.

It's miles too early to be up but it's getting light. Maybe I'll fall asleep now? But already on the other side of the world some friends are waking up. I check them out. We chat. My back is starting to ache and I realise my left leg is sore. Maybe another Sevredol will do the trick? Only one. Be a good boy. It's not long now and the world will soon be awake. But some part of me realises this isn't so. Most people are still deep in sleep.

These are the most beautiful hours – the hours of anticipation. It's going to be another stunningly hot day. Light comes in through blinds and curtains. Everything appears beautiful though my back is sore and when I move my left leg the limb barely refuses to function. So what? I'm alive. Then I remember that nasty little word buried in the report – incurable. But then I say, what does incurable mean? Aren't we all strictly speaking incurable. Nobody gets out of here alive. Maybe it's just that I'm slightly more 'incurable' than others. Can see it more clearly.

It's very beautiful now and I can see out the back window a fume of pink-gold clouds Tintoretto might have been jealous of. Further over is the hard jut of Mt Wellington. There's still at least an hour before I can go and make D's coffee. He sleeps

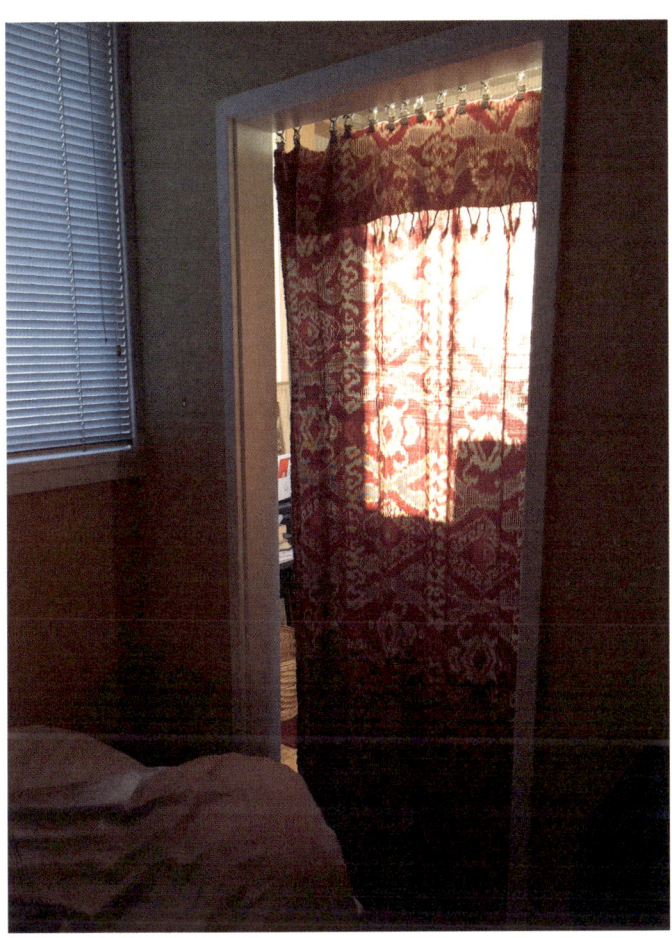

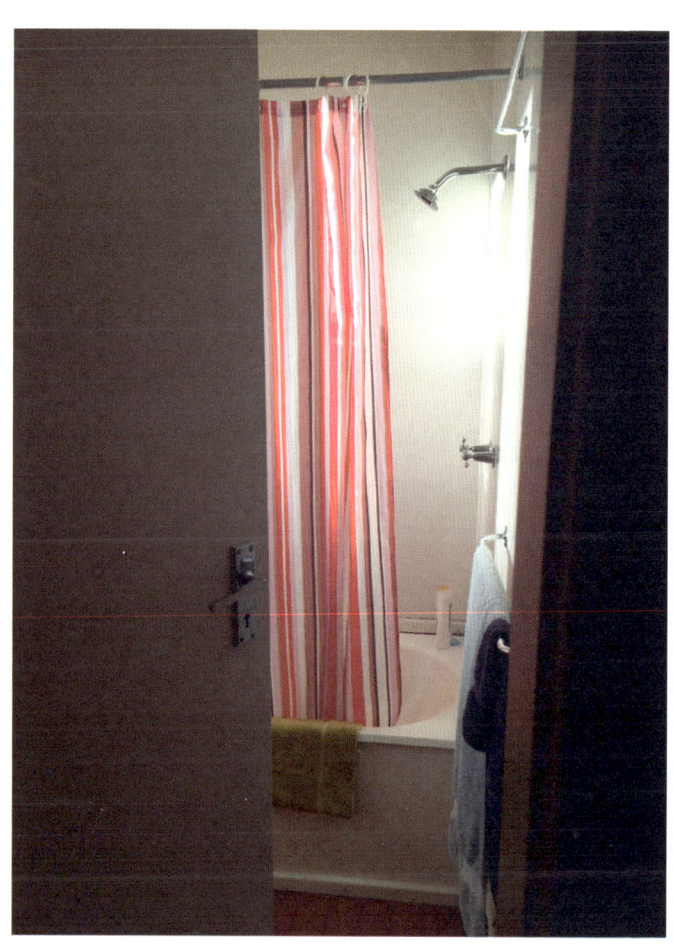

on while I lie here looking around me, thinking, Well that's another night done and dusted and I'm still here. And I know it's only a matter of time before FB starts lighting up and then my day will begin again and people will chat, and soon enough it's the contemporary version of sparrowspark – lots of noise. But just now I lie back on the bed, easing my sore back, and allow myself to enjoy the sheer luxury of being alive.

December 10, 3.17 a.m.

This is my morning breakfast. Twenty pills. Or rather this is what goes with breakfast. At the start I used to try and swallow some of these while eating. Then I made a change in procedure. I decided quaffing the pills was so unpleasant, such an interruption, that they could wait their turn, be exiled to the very end of the meal where, penitentially, I would open my mouth, thrust down the blighters and, accompanied by a big mouthful of water, flush them into my system.

In this way they didn't ruin the whole breakfast. They had their own special moment, over as soon and inoffensively as possible.

Last night I 'forgot' to take my before-bed medication. This led to a sudden irruption into pain in the night. I got up and took the pills, lecturing myself on my inability to accept what had to be accepted: a plethora of pills with every meal, and at the beginning and end of each day, for the foreseeable future.

It's not too much to ask – in fact is very little – but somehow the human bridles at enforced necessity and tries to deviate.

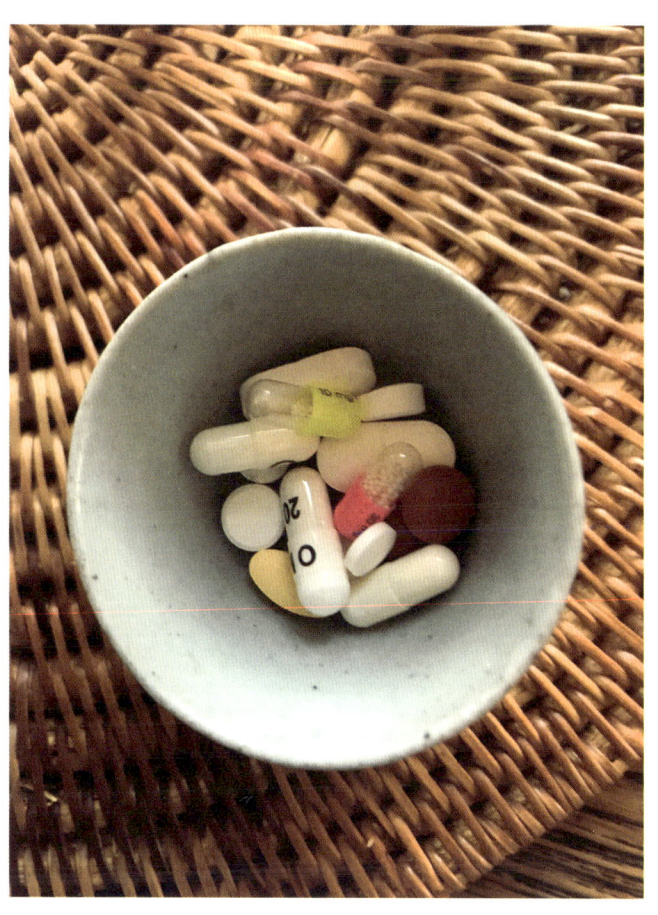

Does it amount to trying to elude the ineluctability of your condition? Yes, probably.

But this is where the small matter of choice – the saving grace of choice – enters the picture. You can change the order in which you do things. You can try and have your say within a limited context of action.

For example: breakfast. It didn't take me long, after beginning my pill regime, to notice a strange taste in my mouth on awakening. Most upsetting, on drinking my first morning cup of tea (breakfast-sized cup, tea a mixture of Lapsang Souchong and Indian leaf tea – brisk, fresh, sharp in flavour, stingingly hot), I experienced a certain deadness – a flatness – in taste. What had happened? The tea was brackish, had no flavour, seemed thin as gruel. It had no punch.

I made a decision: change teas. I now have a heavily scented natural tea – Ginger root and Lemongrass: this hits the taste buds with a nice ping of energy, is very clear and sharp, almost astringent.

I also decided to toast two very thin Vogel slices and smear on butter and Vegemite: an early morning savoury treat. A wild digression of taste, and completely unlike my doormat hospital toast, delivered cold to the door.

But this is a mere entrée to the full fandangle of breakfast, which is porridge soaked overnight with raisins and nuts, complemented this morning by stewed apricots and fresh raspberries. I also had the mad luxury of mango yoghurt. You could say it is a taste overkill. Flagellation of the taste buds in order to experience pleasure.

This is my way of saying I am enjoying eating, I am enjoying food. The pills are exiled like poor relatives standing at the door, able only to watch the feast and await their ignominious moment when they are swallowed without so much as a comment.

And now today an old friend, Mary Trewby, asked D and me round for lunch. Mary made the most extraordinarily sensational range of tasting dishes. Everything bit at the taste buds, frisked the inside of my mouth, assaulted the deadening effects of chemical pills and hustled them out the door with lively, coming-at-ya tastes. I felt thrilled, honoured, sated, blitzed.

There is choice, even in the prison yard of pills.

Later:
A friend said to me he was surprised by my FB posts as I had always been such a private person. I thought about this and I could not say I am sure that person exists anymore. That private self. I said goodbye to him without being aware of it when they wheeled me into Acute Oncology.

As for who this new person is, maybe that is what all these inquiring posts are about. I'm trying to find out.

In the meantime, to escape this quandary, D takes me to the beach. He wrenches me from out of my dark cave and broils my soul on the hot sand . . . and I like it.

December 12, 4.19 a.m.

The humility of my condition. It is only when I approach the cancer clinic I see all the other wanderers and strays either coming away or walking in the same direction. Discreetly one

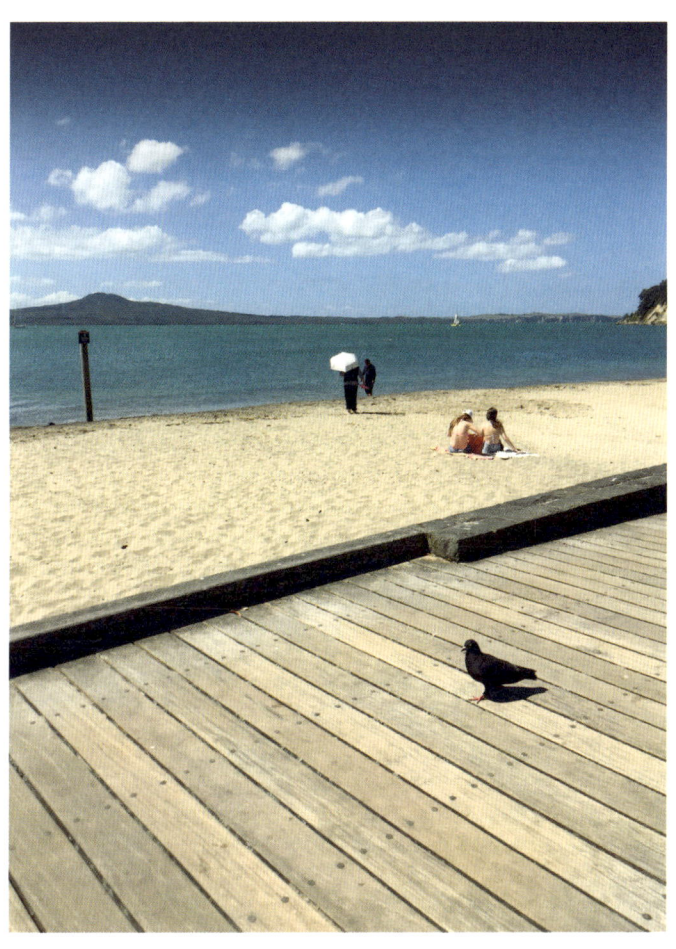

surveys them: are you like me? Do you have a slight impediment to your step? Is your face a little grey? Or do you actually just work here and are passing by? If so, I discount you as a malingerer, unworthy of inspection. I actually feel impatient (irrationally).

Then, inside the waiting room: the anxious couples of all ages. The old ones so familiar with one another no words are needed. Worst of all the young couple with a new baby, a baby so tiny it hardly seems human – it seems like the last drop of human evolution yet clinging on, and the parents desperate, protective, proud, uncertain.

Inside the room where I'll be having chemo in a few weeks: it's empty today and as it's a private facility c/- Southern Cross, the chairs are white vinyl and it has a strange ambience somewhere between country club and nurses' station.

We go through all the possible emergencies and crises and what to look for. I see D's face suddenly look drawn. He has to be vigilant, he has to listen. I try and concentrate, and although I know it's going to happen to me some unreality principle kicks in and all I think about is what wig will I get when my hair falls out on the second chemo. Should I go Andy Warhol? When I mention this to D he doesn't see the joke and remains silent.

We drive home in the heat of mid-December Auckland. Tepid, slightly seething, luxurious if you weren't doing anything. Since I didn't sleep at all well last night I plan a siesta. This doesn't mean I'll sleep, as I know now sleep cannot be willed. Sleep is a gift like laughter. It eludes you when you desperately need it. Then you surrender to it, as in an embrace.

The date is fixed for my first chemo now. Wednesday 10 January 2018 at 1.30 p.m. at the Mercy Hospital, Auckland.

December 13, 2.06 a.m.

The Man Who Shocked the Nation

I'm sorry if this post trespasses on the patience of readers, but just stay with me, or close your eyes and move on.

This is about something you can't stop thinking about when you get sick. It has nothing to do with your illness. But there it is. It just won't go away. (This is the final post I will ever write on the subject.)

My obsession is what a friend enjoyed calling my own personal 'GOFTAGATE'.

After I yelled out 'Fuck off, sexist shit' at John Inman on live television in 1987, I was outed as 'the GOFTA slob' by *Truth* one week later. It led to considerable damage to my career as a film-maker. My name went under a cloud.

Intellectually I stood up for what I had done. I had spoken truth to power. I was used to doing this, protesting about the demolition of Auckland's heritage, for gay rights etc. But subjectively I knew in my heart I had brought shame on the family name. I had been bad mannered, yelling out in public at 'an overseas guest', and even worse had used a four-letter word which was then all but unheard in public discourse.

To most people my anger seemed incomprehensible – what was a sexist shit anyway? What had that nice funny camp fellow done to offend that nasty uptight politico? What business was it of his anyway? This incomprehension framed the whole event. I was never given a chance to explain or frame my argument. My act was so scandalous I had forfeited any right to speak.

In this way I came to represent the entire disastrous night/ event. This just emphasised my powerlessness: my inability to

EXPOSED!

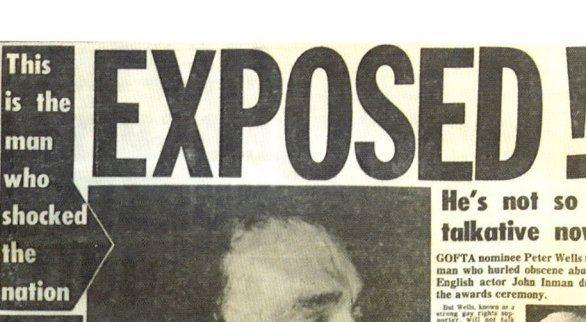

> This
> is the
> man
> who
> shocked
> the
> nation

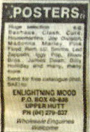

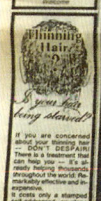

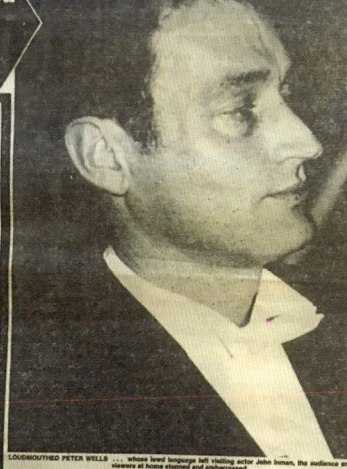

LOUDMOUTHED PETER WELLS ... whose lewd language left visiting actor John Inman, the audience and viewers at home stunned and embarrassed.

He's not so talkative now

GOFTA nominee Peter Wells is the man who hurled obscene abuse at English actor John Inman during the awards ceremony.

But Wells, known as a strong gay rights supporter, will not talk about it in the sober light of day.

When contacted by Truth he said "I'm not going to make a comment" and slammed down the phone.

As Inman came onto the stage Wells — who was nominated for a GOFTA in the best television director category for his work on Jewel's Dart, a story about a transsexual — screamed "sexist slut" for all to hear.

Repeat

Inman didn't quite catch it, or couldn't believe his ears if he did, and asked for a repeat.

As the audience hushed Wells again shouted "sexist slut, I ... off."

It was heard quite clearly by the crowd and the TV audience at home watching the live broadcast. TVNZ have since apologised for this.

Though the audience has been accused of being a rowdy rabble Wells' unnecessary distribe had even the most loutish embarrassed.

Shaken

Inman looked shaken but carried on regardless.

When he's not being rude and insulting overseas guests, Wells is a drama and short story writer, film critic and director.

He wrote the recently shown TV drama A Death in the Family about an AIDS victim

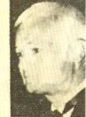

JOHN INMAN ... he had the good grace to ignore the uncouth jeers.

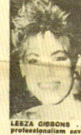

LEEZA GIBBONS ... professionalism saved the day.

and says it was heard the death of a friend last year.

Wells also co-directed the programme.

Directed

In 1981 be directed Foolish Things and in 1983, Little Queen which were both international Film Festival entrants and in 1984 he directed the drama, Being Modern

NON-EVENT OF YEAR

Where were the stars

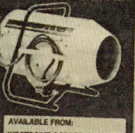

GOSSIP columnist David Hartnell says the GOFTA awards were the "show-business non-event of the year."

"We were promised a star studded evening but where were the stars?"

Hartnell said he was appalled by the loutish treatment of overseas guests Leeza Gibbons and John Inman by a hound up audience.

"Apart from them I don't think I would be able to name six stars who were there.

"That's why I can't write a gossip column about the GOFTA awards.

Hartnell said he couldn't believe the travelogue which introduced the show.

"It was pathetic. Where were all the shots of so-called celebrities getting out of their cars and a commentary of what they were wearing?"

Hartnell also slammed the choice of award presenters.

"Ilona Rodgers was the only one with any class. She could have walked onto the set of Dynasty.

Ridiculous

"It's ridiculous when we've got a designer like Warden Neill here in town who has dressed the stars in Hollywood and

Hartnell also thought the space and style costumes bags Leeza Gibbons and Nic Nolan had to wear were appalling.

"John Inman was right when he said Nic looked like a duvet cover gone wrong.

"And it was insulting to Leeza to make her look like a sued role of tin foil.

over $1000 on the first and they crammed into tables, at least one to many to a table."

The food was hors d'oeuvres and dinner as promised. Hartnell said no two people who sick after eating it.

Restless

"In my opinion just can't do any emotion live on said.

speak, hit back or explain my point of view. Hence these 30 years of at times painful silence and now two posts in which I have tried to think through the 'difficulty of my position'.

I was aware I had wounded my parents because I bore their name and they had had no part in what seemed my showy bad behaviour. That was my most intimate hurt. They had brought me up to be well mannered, courteous and above all kind. But there were hidden tensions. I was always trying to do well to offset what I knew caused them pain – my homosexuality. They were conservative Pākehā, limited in their acquaintance with anyone not heterosexual. I was always trying to over-achieve, to say, 'Look I'm all right. I'm okay, it's all all right.' Then at my most vulnerable moment, as an ambitious 37-year-old-film-maker seemingly on the very point of success, I 'made a fool of myself in front of the nation' and the family name was dragged into the mud.

I remember going out for my weekly meal with them in Mt Eden the following week. Not a word was said; there was no hint of reproach or bewilderment. There was just a depth of silence which was, in fact, their version of kindness.

I see that now. I was infinitely relieved not to be questioned, or accused, or asked what on earth I thought I was doing. Instead we ate our meal modestly, quietly, as if there was literally nothing to say.

It was many years later I began to connect my father's increased drinking to his sense of humiliation at the way I had exposed myself in public – as a loud-mouthed, opinionated homosexual who thought his views were so important everyone had to hear about them. (Not that I thought that precisely. I saw it entirely differently: I was standing up for minority rights and the ability for LGBTQI people to speak in their own voice, through drama, at a time when this was not accepted as valid.)

I had such a vivid sense of Dad's presence on the night of the GOFTAS. He was always 'second best' in my mother's eyes. He had failed to deliver the social status that she believed was hers by right. This was never said, but it was something known in that quiet unreality known as family life. That night when I didn't win the prizes I had perhaps thought I might have, I felt Dad's ghost standing so close to me he was almost palpable.

'You will never be good enough,' he said. He turned to me and recognised me, and I knew I would never be good enough either.

So all that over-achieving to placate my parents, to soothe them, to persuade them I was, yes, homosexual but my life was fine – I saw in this instance that I had failed too, and this was part of my devastation. I will never be good enough, either.

I don't think that now, but its shadow lay over my life for quite a few years. I lost my self-esteem. I doubted myself. The taint still stayed with me, like a bad taste in my mouth. I knew to malicious people I would always be someone who made a fool of himself in public (regardless of the very real issues of representation and misrepresentation). It took me a long while to free myself from this taint, to recognise it was a disastrous incident in which I was implicated. Besides, time shunted me forward. I was always thinking, always full of ideas – making films, then writing books; along with Stephanie Johnson I began to hatch a plan for a properly professional writers' festival for Auckland.

And in the end, at some point (like now when I am sick and have limited time to put my house in order), it becomes one to leave a wounding past behind.

That the scandal – the hurt – is still so alive to me now, 30 years later, is what amazes me. Dad died in late 1987 and my mother left me in April this year. I could wound them no longer. Yet GOFTAGATE still flared up into my consciousness with all the heat of the wronged, the maligned, the unjustly treated. Coming to terms with GOFTA has been part of my coming to terms with mortality. I want to make all plain and truthful.

I was very angry when I did not win any prizes, and an incredible fury built up in me and exploded when the 'acceptable homosexual identity' (i.e. someone who could never say what they were but could act out the campest caricature – a heterosexual projection) was welcomed on to the stage. I had directed and co-written a trans drama that was made not in 2016 or 2017 in New York or LA but in 1986 in Aotearoa New Zealand. It was a drama which also starred a trans actor, Georgina Beyer, in a role which led to her being a finalist in the Best Women Actor category – itself a breakthrough. It was a big leap forward, a nod to a distant future. But in terms of a NZ drama award, it was judged 'not good enough'. It was not equal to TVNZ product. And then I had to countenance that withering stereotype, that personification of everything inauthentic you could humanly imagine at the time of the AIDS crisis – a man who cannot even say who he is – emerging on the stage to applause.

That is when I opened my mouth and my fury poured out. At the time it seemed part of a chaotic molten event – I suppose you could call it a 'live' event in the truest sense. It never occurred to me there was no sound delay, nor that the peculiarities of recorded sound would pick up my voice and project it with such force. When John Inman asked me to repeat what I said – I can't recall his exact words but it was along the lines of 'I can't hear what you're saying, sweetie' – I took up my call with renewed force.

In that moment all my fury at being a second-class citizen, at not having equal rights, at having to fight for any legitimacy – all the pain right back to the wounds of the playground, a life lived in inequality – exploded through my mouth – out my throat. (The phenomenon is called 'Velvet Rage' – this is from a book subtitled 'Overcoming the Pain of Growing Up Gay in a Straight Man's World'.) Was I in fact trying to scream down the patriarchy?

At the time it seemed part of the blazing drunken energy of the night: there was almost no food but endless cheap Australian champagne. I had no idea I had caused a scandal. It was only days later that it became apparent I was trapped in one.

A friend rang me up and said to go down to my local dairy. I walked down to the local shop in Grey Lynn, saw the billboard outside on the street. I bought the scandal rag with shaking hands and opened it to a page with a photograph of me in white tie and tails – a rather sedate, composed-looking person, I thought. I was named.

That was the real start of the scandal – the hunting of the slob.

I have already outlined what happened: the vendetta, the slowing down of a career, the 'friends' who vanished. The horrible phone calls. The filthy notes. My self-doubt was probably worst of all. Had I done wrong?

In the end, for my sanity, I had to turn my back on this particular part of my past and move on.

Until now when its evil genie arose again, casting the

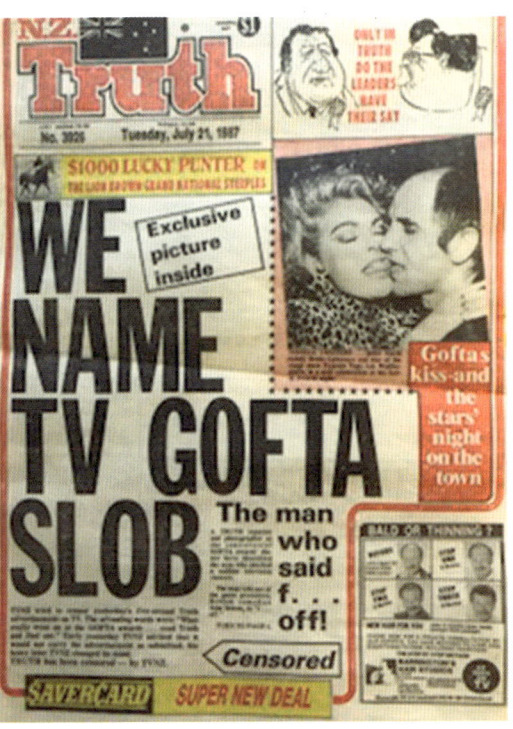

authenticity of my life into shade. As I became sicker I had this desire 'to set the record straight'.

Then, and it is part of the living 'interconnectivity' of what I'm doing here – writing in a public medium like FB – an acquaintance, a friend, got in touch.

'Your post took me right back,' Fiona Samuel wrote to me in a comment on my first GOFTA post. 'I was on the GOFTA Board, representing Actors Equity, and when John Inman was mooted as a presenter I said our members would not welcome it, for the same reason you didn't. The Writers Guild rep said so too. We were firmly put in our places by the TVNZ producer responsible for the show, who told us we were "up ourselves" (practically worst sin in NZ) and that his "old mother in name of suburb redacted" LOVED John Inman and that's the kind of audience he cared about, not arty farty wankers who can't take a joke. So he was warned but chose not to listen.'

Fiona went on to warn the TVNZ producer about the impossibly complex four-tier prize system in which some winners could come to the podium to speak, others could accept an award but not speak, while others again got their award at the table (saving travel time) but actually were able to speak, while Category D winners, 'the lowest of the low', would be given their awards at the table, 'the remains of their vile dinner all around them'. They could not speak.

It led to a Marx Brothers level of anarchy on the night, 'with nobody knowing what to do, the winners stopped confused – floor managers were actually lying on the floor [trying to wave people either on to the podium or back to their seats according to the shots that had been pre-planned] – everyone wondering what had happened? It was excruciating,' she commented. 'I was 26 and there in a raggedy but beautiful deep blue lace dress and an old military jacket, watching in amazement as this slow motion horror show unfolded.'

It was the year of the infamous space-age set, with flashing lights that led to epileptic attacks among New Zealand viewers. If this midsummer's madness and chaos was not enough, 'on the morning of the awards, the board was informed that the chief executive (i.e. only paid employee) had absconded with thousands of dollars of embezzled funds and no one knew how the dreadful bunfight was now to be paid for . . .'

'I'm so sorry, but not surprised, to hear you were pilloried for your outburst of honesty,' Fiona wrote. She ended by saying: 'I was so glad you shouted out – I felt vindicated in my "up-yourself-ness" and secretly took you for a friend.'

This touched me deeply.

Fiona's vivid account helped me to understand the 'slow motion horror show' on another level too. For too long it had seemed to be my own personal shame. I could never adjust my sense of myself as someone polite, empathetic, and who valued kindliness as one of the most important virtues, to the public representation of me as a loudmouthed slob who had 'ruined' a public event by shouting out obscenities. Which one was I? Or was I the person who 'would never be good enough really', a failure of some kind – invited to the feast but metaphorically turned away at the door? Or was I none of these things, more elusive, perpetually trying to find his way forward to a kind of personal truth while acknowledging some of the damage of the past?

Fiona had helped me bracket the GOFTA night, understand it, widen the lens so I finally did understand. The event was an unmitigated disaster on nearly every front. The choice of John Inman, at the very least, was politically insensitive to the point of being provocative during the heated agitation for Homosexual Law Reform and the agony of ever-worsening AIDS statistics. It was an insult to every LGBTQI person trying to live an authentic life at that most challenging of times.

I was too nervously attached to social and political change. It wasn't simply 'a drama' I was representing in a film I'd felt sure would win a prize, so much as a point of view, a right to establish our legitimate presence as part of NZ life, as seen through the prism of drama.

Fiona ended her post: 'You were entirely right and history is on your side.

So this is the spot where at long last I bury the GOFTA Slob. He has silently accompanied me for far too long. Stolen into my dreams and thieved away my rest. Given me a false identity that made me doubt my own reality. I did make a mis-step. It would have been better if I had remained silent. But I did not, and I lived – painfully at times – with the consequences. Yet time is long and it is the irony of the situation that I ended up being the one person carrying the burden of a memory which others had long since divested as 'so much rubbish', a silly event, a meaningless mess of a night.

I do not have the time any more to carry GOFTA's weight – its dross. I do not have the energy – so at the end of this sentence I divest it into space –

There is a kind of beauty in sleeplessness but it's a seductive, poisonous beauty. (It's possible I'm sleepless now simply because I'm not physically active enough in the day.) But my mind is also very alert. It won't stop. This is despite the fact I prepare my nest – the large single bed in which I now sleep – lovingly. I have my books nearby, an unrealistic number of them – as if somehow in the middle of the night I might want to 'change trains'. All those queued-up sentences like so many trains waiting to enter a station are my friends. I might need them at a lonely, perilous hour.

There is my large bottle of water and a crystal glass. (I often wake up with a caked mouth so dry it causes me to panic. Pills, I guess.) There is my iPhone of course which is utterly essential. It makes me feel 'I am never alone' (rightly or wrongly).

(Often on my phone I will sketch out a future post for FB then send it in an email to myself. Somehow the dark intransigence of night seems so suitable for this sketching out, amending, changing.)

But it's more than that. I consciously chose good cotton sheets and pillow cases once I knew I would spend a lot of time in bed. D bought me some cracking cotton pyjamas, the first pyjamas I have owned since I was a child. (I am reminded of Steph Johnson saying to me when she was a child and often having operations on her legs and feet she was always allowed to wear her own pyjamas in hospital and how much this meant to her – a sort of body within a body.)

So I have these beautiful sheets within which to lie. Pillows of course, plus the essential small cushion to wedge against my troublesome hip. Drugs to wipe away pain, if it gets bad.

And on top of the bed I have placed a wool rug. I'd forgotten how comforting a wool rug can be. During the day, even a warm day, I can lie down under a wool rug and have a snooze. It takes me back to a Plunket boyhood, I guess, to my capable mother, to being looked after.

This is all by way of prep for sleep each night.

I always go to bed eagerly. But somehow it happens – during the long lockdown – that time runs away from me and ceases to be so friendly. It tightens round me and I become aware of both a solitariness and also a kind of quizzing, almost corrosive sensibility. So how are you really? might be the question. Or are you really coping or just putting up a public façade? You can cry with self-pity at these times: no one will see or hear you. Thank god. The night continues on in its seemingly endless, pitiless projection of itself. It's particularly hard between 3 a.m. and 4.30 a.m.

Yet the fact is, at daybreak I feel a most improbable optimism. I can't explain it. Is it for having endured, and survived, another long silent night? Or is it that I understand, empathise and even approve of the dazzling beauty of sleeplessness, just as I understand its potency is towards evil, or at least destructiveness. How much sleeplessness can one person take? Or am I just unwakingly awake?

Yet the fact is last night I plunged down the deepest shaft of sleep the moment I put my head on the pillow. This was the evening I finally finished talking about GOFTA. It had been a more intense process than I could ever have imagined. So many messages from FB friends came through it had a living, enveloping quality. Gradually I began to understand that the nightmare of the incident was over. I saw I had tortured myself too long. I slept the sleep of someone who had travelled a vast

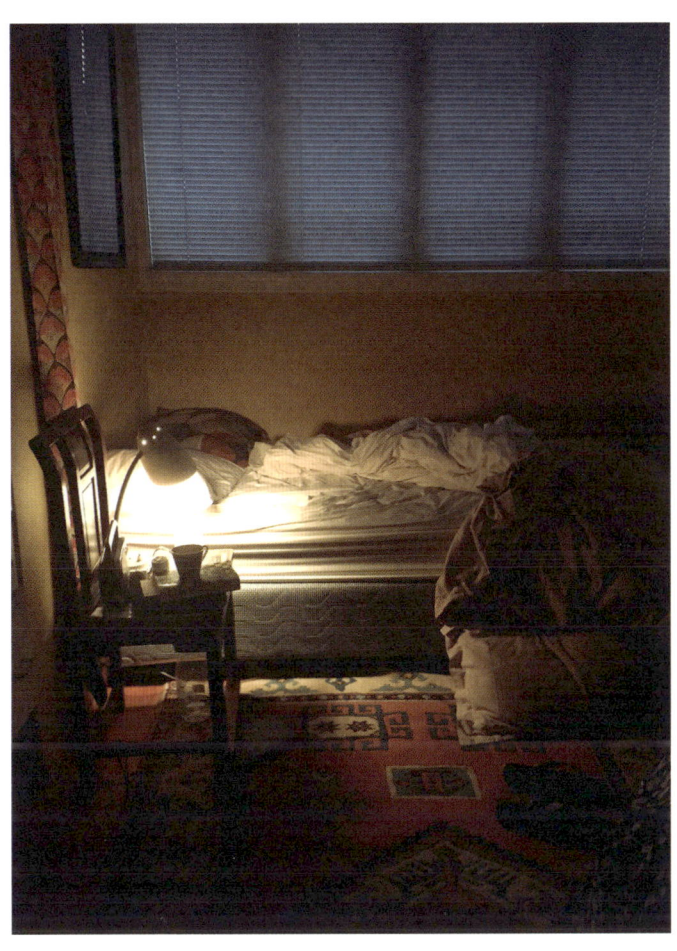

distance, as if I had walked from my 37th year right into the skin and body of the man I am now. I felt in a state of grace.

Then – in the early hours of the morning – as if in a dream I began to hear rain falling . . .

December 15, 5.04 a.m.

FB is addictive and I have become addicted to its likes and comments – they have become my crutches on which I struggle along. But to what degree is my self-portrait real – to what degree a willed portrait, a sketch, leaving out certain melancholy facts which nobody wants to know? To what degree is the whole exercise based on voyeurism, boredom, my own exhibitionism and narcissism – a desire to display, even when in the most moribund circumstances. Besides, you are borrowing the plumage of KM (Katherine Mansfield). She wants it back.

'A patient' was how I saw myself described in a nurse's notes, and I thought to myself how valid – patient as in endless time, patient as in passive, patient as in abidingly awaiting what will happen to me. It was only when I googled metastatic cancer that I saw, with a shudder, it was called stage 4 cancer. Is there a stage beyond?

Where am I on this spectrum of patience and impatience? Is it meant to be bad for morale for 'a patient' to grasp that they will die sooner or later? And where am I? Incurable but with a chance to live at least a further 18 months – that is the promise of chemo, radiation and hormone treatment? But beyond that: 'I've known men in your situation who've lived many, many years – almost twenty.' These are verbal assurances which I suck up instantly in my need for affirmation. Nobody knows, nobody can tell us the truth. Hence this need for patience.

Later:
Looking round the room last night I realised we, old friends tried and true, were all roaring with laughter at the same moment. It was like an apotheosis of glee, a gust of hilarity that overtook us in one gigantic sneeze.

Why? Were we all suddenly granted the consciousness that we were lucky to be alive, lucky to be together in one room, lucky to occupy a schism of time and place? There we all were laughing into infinity, gloriously happy, and it seemed to me I had never seen such happy people, determined in that second to outface risk, accidents, happenstance, bad luck, and to spend everything, all we had, laughing at fate.

Then the second passed and we returned to ourselves and I knew I had seen something secret, something wonderful – right into the heart of friendship.

December 17, 3.59 a.m.

How do you mediate between your anxieties, your expectations and the realities of what a medical intervention can do? That's the hard – or is it the best? – bit: your own personal response to medications which have their well-described side-effects. What is the reality? How will it turn out for me?

These thoughts are prompted by a new medication I'm taking. I'm starting a course of hormones called Zoladex.

Its aim is to neutralise the testosterone which is feeding my cancer, causing it to metastasise (was there ever an uglier verb?)

There are many issues to do with this intervention which profoundly disturb me. These are just some of the side-effects one could expect. The creation of breasts. Hot flushes. Loss of sexual appetite. Loss of erection. Fatness in the face. Cloudy thought. Depression.

Yet even beyond the core terror of 'will I be me?' there are other issues to do with responsiveness.

Some old friends got in touch. Terry has prostate cancer too. He and his partner Peter briefed me on what to expect with chemo. But when we got to the Zoladex injection Terry warned me that it might hurt. Imagination is four-fifths of the equation with me. I began to fear getting the needle.

As it was, my kindly doctor put on some local anaesthetic and before I knew it I felt a metallic presence in my gizzard pushing through. For one moment I felt fear – a child's fear of a needle – but then I relaxed and it was over.

Part of me is a coward in apprehension. Another part of me is shamelessly insistent on being an eye witness.

Am I calling back on the strength of my ancestors? Is this the payback for my close attendance on my almost 101-year-old mother before she died?

It wasn't that she was brave, it was just there was a human eloquence in the way she bore witness to the things that were happening to her – there was an element of good grace. She was an old Pākehā woman who was used to not complaining, to taking things as they came, of not grandstanding. Maybe she even had some inner strength to withstand, to survive.

I'm not sure, as I know towards the end she was also quite childish about pain, exaggerating it – but then it is quite possible she felt things more keenly as her strength gave out. Her skin was thin, her end near. She returned to being the little girl she was at the beginning – someone I had never seen.

It seems strange to me I was given the gift – or debt – of being such a close eye witness to her getting ready for death. (I'm talking March–April this year.) Yet was it this that prepared me to have a relatively steady gaze at what happened to me so quickly after she died? If anything prepared me, it was seeing her go through her own preparations for departure – a mother I loved deeply but whose care had exhausted me and worn me to the bone.

Do I feel her beside me now? Not profoundly – not in a kind of 'you are in the same room with me now' kind of way. But yes, I feel her presence as if in another slightly distant but still coeval room. Does this help me? Yes.

As for my own individual experience of what lies ahead – the mystery that is future tense. I have my improbable optimism, the source of which I cannot diagnose. I have the reality of the seriousness of my complaint – a diagnosis of metastatic prostate cancer that is not curable. How the two relate (my body and the disease) is perhaps dependent on my response towards medical interventions, my biography. And some further mysterious part which no human can name.

This (page 76) is a photo of my mother in her 101st year. I was sitting with her and she closed her eyes. I put my iPhone on silent and photographed her. To me she looks exhausted by the business of staying alive, but there is also some inalienable dignity about her which to me amounts to beauty.

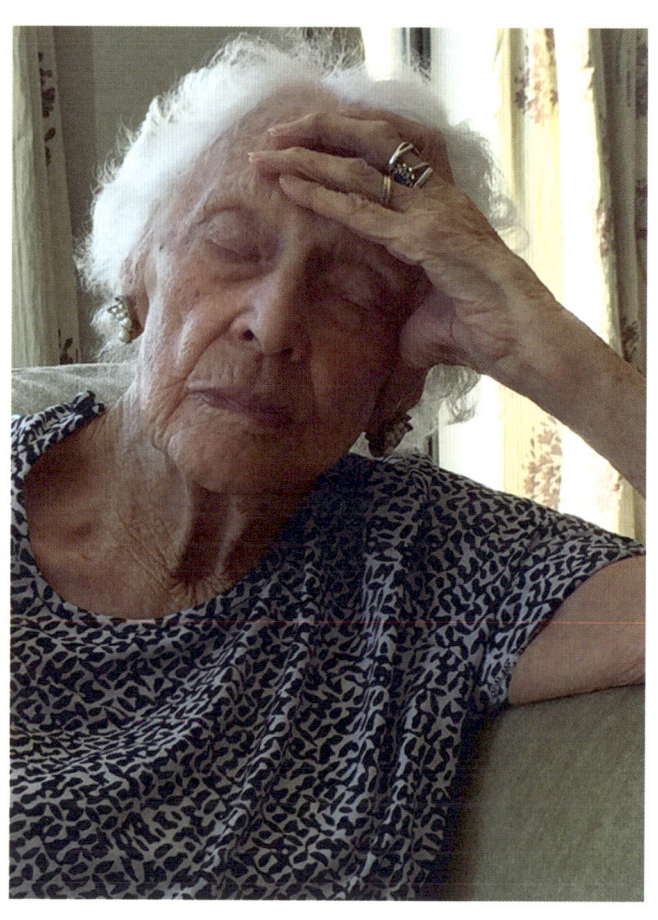

December 18, 1.25 a.m.

Zoladex frightens me.

'Most men lose their sex drive and have erection difficulties during hormonal therapy.' This is big stuff for me – for any man. My desire is being taken away from me, medically removed in order that I have a better chance of staying alive.

'You may gain weight, particularly around your waist.' 'You may experience mood swings.' 'Some men become low in mood or depressed after taking Zoladex for several months.' 'You may notice changes in your memory or ability to concentrate.'

I'm usually inured to all the cluster of negativities that are part and parcel of contemporary medicine. But this . . . this is something entirely new, something that challenges some essential part of myself, the core of being me.

Sex, sexuality, desire has played such a transformative role in my whole life that to face this now, at such a late stage, is somehow baffling, both frightening – how will I react? – will sexual feelings ever come back? And confronting. Who will I be without desire? What will I be? Will I even be me?

Or is this the last barter of the desperate? 'It may be used to control prostate cancer in men whose cancer has spread to other parts of the body (advanced or metastatic prostate cancer.)'

It frightens the fuck out of me – perhaps more literally than I know.

I'm living through so many changes now. But this is a big one, a very big one. Is it the biggest of all – the removal of want? Will I keep looking, being amazed, sometimes saddened, other times bedazzled by the sheer never-ending effrontery which is desire? Want. That fundamental needy word in which all is made explicit. I want. You want. A want of kindness. A want to be touched, loved, valued. Validated. Want. Endless want. Till the grave, I suspect.

Or in this case till the hormone lessens my masculinity, my love of the mystery of male beauty, till I become some kind of neuter. Will I still be me in that quiescent state? Or am I already maybe 'not me' as the sickness changes me into somebody else?

It's not like my body has lost its materiality. In many ways it's still there, though it's lost its elasticity from too much stasis and bed rest. But as for that obsessive cleaving need. It has already been lessened by my taking hormones in pill form. Now it's an injection which lasts one month. Others are to follow.

My whole life has been defined by my sexual preference, once it became readable to myself and other people. For better or for worse. It became who I was, it gelled around me, and slowly I became my sexual preference and that was how I 'identified' and saw the world. Because of my age – when I was born – I became 'gay'. I was 'out'. I was to a degree transparent as to what and who I was. I was a lover of male beauty, of swelling chests and muscular legs, of a certain kind of masculine charm, even vigour. Maleness was my musk, my magic, my muse. This all happened without my thinking or inclination. It just was. It didn't stop me having close friends who were heterosexual, male, female, trans. I was eclectic, I liked difference just as I liked humour, elegance, irony, Old Sheffield Plate and people who listened carefully before they replied. Beauty wasn't skin deep; it was everywhere if you knew where to look for it.

Like many gay men who had had a traumatic passage through youth in the 1950s I was late arriving at the party.

I only felt safe opening myself to rapturous sex as an adult. I had been more than lucky to have a faithful lover who loved me. It was more than I deserved. And now this whole astonishing platter is being taken to a side window in a high-rise building, and scurfed off like so much rubbish you have to get rid of, just so you can survive in the most elemental – vegetative – way possible. Just so you can stay alive.

Atul Gawande, in *Being Mortal*, quoting Ronald Dworkin: 'Whatever the limits and travails we face, we want to retain the autonomy – the freedom – to be the authors of our lives. This is the very marrow of being human . . . all we ask is to be allowed to remain the writers of our own story. [But] that story is ever changing.'

Changes.
1.
My body has changed shape. I now have a large and swollen abdomen above my hips. It has become impossible to keep my pants on when I walk along on my crutches. Several times I have had to choose between grabbing my pants before they fall down off my hips or holding on to my crutches. This can happen in the middle of the road. There is nothing for my belt to hold on to any longer. I have had to get braces as the only way to keep my pants on in public.
2.
I was always too ladylike to fart in public. But now I am on a daily medicine to ensure I do not get constipation, which is a side-effect to the daily ingestion of morphine. But the medicine, small brown pills daily, often has the effect that I have to run to the loo, followed by a loud arpeggio of farts that trails away like smoke from the funnel of a coal-burning steamer. I am

no longer ashamed but laugh at the frightful and shameless indecency of my body. It has betrayed a lifetime of manners.
3.
I like 'spending the time of day' with strangers in shops and on the streets – people with whom I suddenly seem to have a lot in common. This is a very surprising development. Before I was always too shy to talk with strangers, but these days I light up if I see someone to chat to. I like everything about it, the inconsequentiality, the not knowing where it will lead, the feeling of universal goodwill. I think this is an outcome of being in hospital, which is a kind of universalising experience, a humbling experience in which you return to being a body. You are stripped down to the essence of being human.
4.
Though on the contrary sometimes I am full of dark malevolence and fury and could curse the human race to perdition. There's no in-between.

Regard this as a report hurriedly written on the run. I have not thought like this for a long time. Before this, I had been too immersed in desire, love, sex to take a step back. I am not taking a step back here so much as having the step taken from me. I don't feel self-pity, only a sense of uncertainty. I do not even, at the moment, feel regret. I am just palpitating this new condition.

Already I feel less interested in sex, even in male beauty. It draws my eye, it does not draw my breath.

Gawande: 'That is why betrayals of the body and mind that threaten to erase character and memory remain among our most awful tortures. The battle of being mortal is the battle to maintain the integrity of one's life – to avoid being so diminished or dissipated or subjugated that who you are becomes disconnected from who you were or wanted to be.'

I do want to live. Of course. But I also want to be me. I want to remain the author of my life. I have fought so hard for the freedom of my sexual identity that it seems an irony that, at this very late moment, I come to a counter, like in a war zone, where I have to hand in my 'uniform', which is taken away, and instead I put on this night dress . . . and I find a bench and I go and lie down . . . and I wait . . .

And there's not only Zoladex. Chemo lies ahead. I sometimes think of Gawande's advice that some people live longer without chemo, enjoy more 'quality of life'. Medicine becomes a gamble in the end. Which treatment? When? Why? And to what end?

And who will I be at the end of it?

Will I still be me?

Later:

D has become obsessed with fitness and dieting. He looks tremendous. I enjoy having this trim stranger inside the house, his muscular legs and taut chest. I am not sure I precisely know him and we have not had 'the talk' about sex, or how we are now at different parts of the clock: me starting to take serious hormones and lose any desire that I have: me with my already wasted body with loss of muscle tissue, the vanishing arse which is really just a series of sad pleats: while he is robust, tanned, has started swimming, goes to the gym for hours. But he bears a face tightened by unhappiness, an inward glance of resentment. I was always a dud deal, I guess. He loves me but resents the curve of fate, its implacable shape – if indeed it is implacable.

I myself go through moods which change from 'This is a theatrical set of circumstances I am emotionally occupying, a kind of role' to 'I can't get away from something that imprisons me' to 'This is a daydream, a very strange one, from which someday I will awaken.' I move between these states on an irregular basis, most of it dependent on mood, what is happening to my body – my level of pain – or maybe just taking a holiday in denial, you know, like going to the pictures. Reality is sometimes just too hard.

December 19, 4 p.m.

Every Christmas when I was a child in Point Chevalier you would hear the sprinkle of a bike bell and see a kid sprinting along on a shiny new bike, his or her face a mask of glee, in a fury of possession, chasing the wind and as happy as a human could ever be.

Imagine my mixed feelings when I turned the corner by our front door and found I had been presented with a shiny new iridescent-green 'walker' by 'Environmental Health Management Services Ltd', completely gratis.

My humiliation at having to rely on an old person's conveyance met with a fillip of excitement, a wild rash of joy, that it would increase my mobility, I could actually go for 'walks' on my own – I could carry shopping – I need no longer hobble and lurch.

Of all the things I most regret about my situation the worst is losing the proud ability to stroll, or amble. Or walk quickly

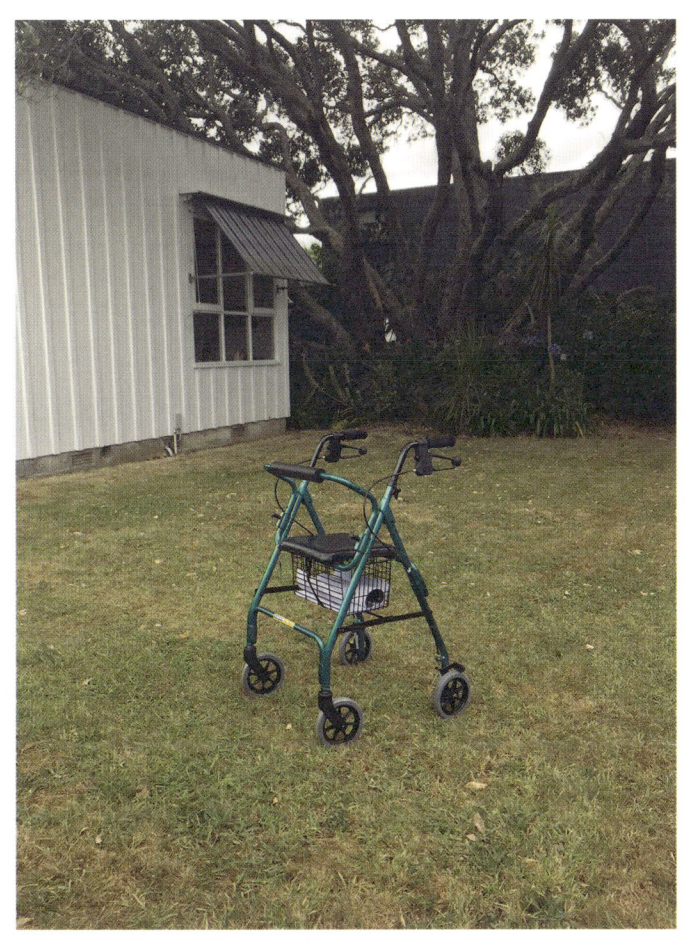

or even run. So to suddenly be presented with this new way of being mobile literally brings tears to my eyes. Okay, some of it is chagrin, humiliation, the hard spell of pride. But I have learnt nothing is more immaterial in this situation than pride. I can no longer afford it. That purse is empty or perhaps always had a hole in its bottom anyway.

I will be like those kids at Pt Chev who used to practise in private, in the back yard, trying to stay upright on their new bikes before brandishing forth on the streets, their faces proud and solemn as spears, everything contained in the juggling act of staying upright.

So I will practise in private the runes of a man on a walker who is walking on air.

Salut to Environmental Health Management Services Ltd and to a health system which is still functioning and which delivers a week before Christmas such a devastating surprise. I am truly deeply grateful and touched. When you see me on my walker just remember I am walking on air.

December 22, 3.34 a.m.

Opening the door to this very atmospheric house in Napier, I suddenly saw it as if for the first time.

It had never seemed more evident than that this house and its bewitching interior (especially on a warm still night) was an expression of love between the two of us. D with his expert eye and extraordinary degree of knowledge had created something personal as a statement, lyrical as a song, a form of identity he

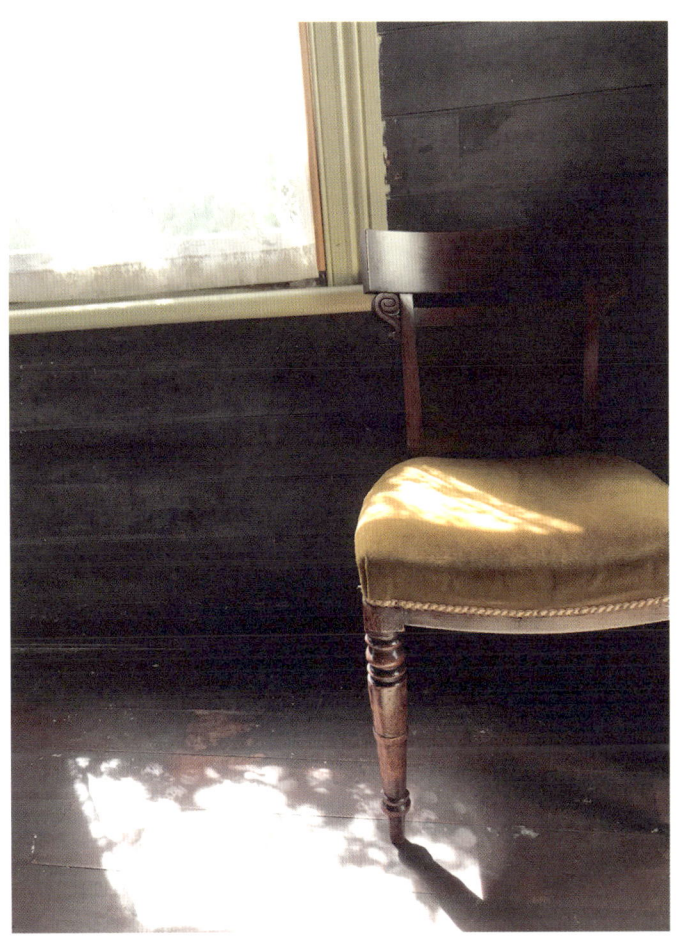

offered to me almost in the form of a dreamworld, yet practical as a place we could live side by side with one another and be content.

Like all relationships, especially one over almost three decades, we had pushed, pulled, fought, argued, had silences and disagreements. Yet I had always known the strength of his love which if anything has grown stronger – though more practically tested – by what is taking place now.

Lately I had begun to worry about him. He seemed exhausted and depressed while I struggled to maintain some equilibrium. He has to stand to the side and offer endless encouragement and practical help while the larger questions – how long do I live, will our relationship ever be as it was, will it keep developing – hover over our heads. (He is over a decade younger than me.) I realise other things – the pills make me garrulous and argumentative at times, intolerant of delays. I keep strange hours in my head. And now that my treatment will be entirely up in Auckland, it creates the question of what will we do with 'the Napier house' – a place I love, feel at home in and which has the additional responsibility of two female cats of some maturity and dependence.

This is the hidden question (just one of them) that lies behind our presence here 'back home' in Napier. Yet at the moment all I hear is the endless fall of silence, the gorgeousness of room after room filled with items, each one personally thought about, looked at, meditated on and chosen, and I suddenly realise how deeply personal this house is. It is a habitat of love, a shelter we had made together as personal as a sentence, as binding as a wedding ring.

Was I lucky or unlucky? I no longer asked that question. I only thought I was lucky to be alive, and to be alive is to try to solve problems, even those that are by their nature insoluble, or perhaps implacable might be a better way to put it. But was I lucky to have D as a partner? I could not have survived the past month without him. I was lucky, I was unlucky, I was a loser and I was a winner too.

I gave the above to Douglas to read and to my surprise he replied as follows:

> Peter
> I value my privacy and I wish to retain my dignity through our current private difficulties, therefore I don't wish to have my current emotional state and or behaviour turned into fodder for social media hangers on.
> So just to make myself very clear – DO NOT mention me or post any images of me at all on Facebook or Instagram under any circumstances.
> Douglas

This puts me in a dilemma as our lives, especially at the moment, are so interwoven.

December 23, 1.22 a.m.

I'm always a little anxious around this part of December. I was trying to think today where and when my ambiguous feelings about Christmas came from.

I think it grew and feasted on all the days our family tried so hard to be like all the other families and failed so abysmally. We always seemed to have tense days. It was a day in which an argument always arrived on cue, like a migraine or like a smashed crystal dish. We did try. Christmas after Christmas we all tried so hard to make it work. Presents, a special something at dinner. But it never worked. All that trying probably meant it was just about impossible for us to relax and enjoy ourselves.

I can, I think, trace it all back to one particular Christmas when it really went wrong. I don't need to go back there but it set a pattern we could never move beyond. It stayed with us, haunting us, quietly freaking us out like a body we all knew was buried under the floorboards until the family dismantled itself.

First of all Dad died in 1987, then almost as an afterthought and too quickly, my handsome and super-bright brother Russell walked into the sky – he was dead at 41 – and this left just Mum and me curating a day we pretty much wished would disappear. Bess and I coped in our own rather dry, amused way, putting Christmas in between quotation marks. Bess could never get used to this 'Christmas' though. It meant she was always aware she had two gay sons and she saw all around her . . . absences mainly – the grandchildren she would never have, the daughters-in-law to improve and fight with, the in-laws she always planned to look down on. There was such a ghostly absence of people who should have been there that it was hard for me to, well, account for myself as me. I always felt a slim minus in this situation, no matter how happy I was with my life, first with Stewart as a partner and then with Douglas. All I could hear was the sad rustle of ghosts.

Of course we didn't treat it as a tragedy and had especially strong gins and tonics which loosened our tongues, but it was still unavoidable – and when those thoughtless gabby bitches

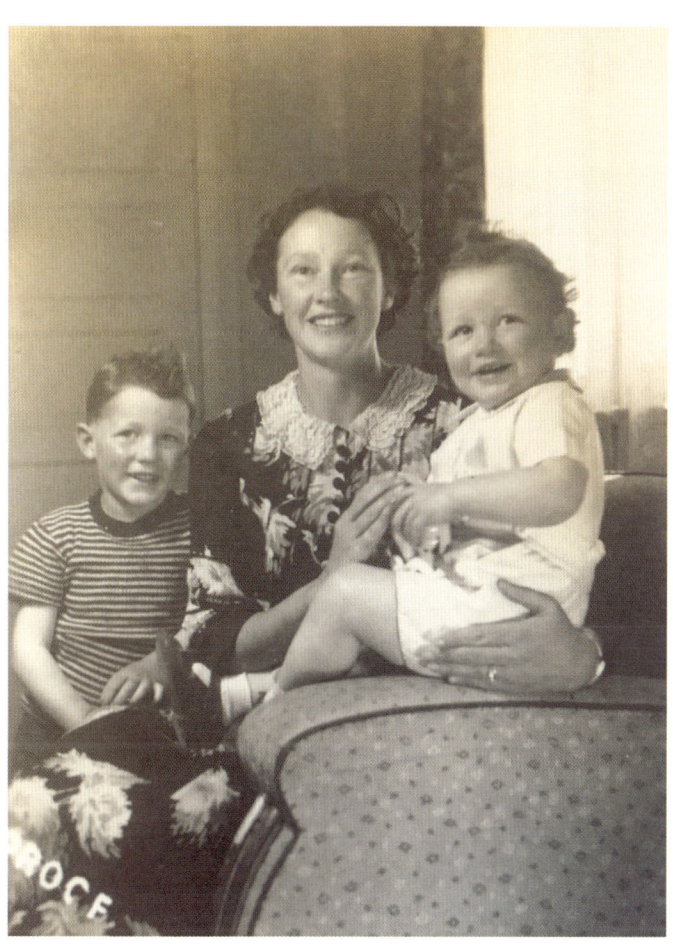

got on the phone and screeched out, 'We had 43 people sitting down at table . . .' I always felt my mother's singular predicament. She could only say, drily, 'Well, there was just Pete and me . . . but we enjoyed ourselves . . .' The rustle of ghosts was always particularly quiet when she said that, I think in sympathy.

It took me many years to shake off these ghosts. It still takes me a conscious effort to relocate myself in the present and accept Christmas can be, well, whatever you want it to be. Like this Christmas, I'll spend it with Douglas, and in the evening we'll join our lovely friend Annie at her splendid house where we'll have a swim in her pool if it's warm enough, then casually barbecue something scrumptious and be low key and relaxed. The following day friends arrive to stay and this is when Christmas kicks off, with people coming and going, friends looping back through time into the past, tying us to the present and the future.

I wish sometimes I went out and bought a Christmas tree and fairy lights and got one of those things you hang on the front door. It would be novel to experience a Christmas in that sort of formatted way – like I was a refugee learning the customs of the country I've newly come to live in. I have learnt to be relaxed about this rather difficult day now – I've learnt not to cart the corpse of my old feelings into the present. But is it a day I look forward to with childish anticipation? Not really.

December 25

The silver hair brush. When my mother Bess got married three months into WW2, she was given all the presents that a middle-class woman of the era could expect. But many were quite modest, like a good-quality travel rug. An exception was the three-piece sterling mirror brush and comb set, each piece stylishly engraved with the initials, interestingly, of her maiden name (BPN) rather than her new married name.

As a child I always liked looking at the elegance of the engraving. Today it is a lost art but at that time any jeweller could produce a fanferol of lettering, each letter curved and with a kind of added dash, like a trumpet blast.

The silver set sat on her dressing table amid a clutter of other bridal crystal, perfume bottles, little boxes to hold jewellery. Yet I don't particularly remember Mum using the brush and comb set – it was set aside for 'best' or for show or for when the Queen happened to drop by for tea, which at that moment in time everyone kind of expected.

It was only when she got older she started using the brush. And of course by that stage the brush was old too. Its bristles were yellow and brittle, but there was enough of the brush left to be useful in tidying up Bess's increasingly thin hair.

In fact as she got older still, the brush was like a scalp massage. In her nineties, then into her hundreds, it was a special pleasure for me to get the old brush and very carefully, very slowly, brush her hair. She might close her eyes or grow silent. Speech was no longer necessary. After I'd finish she might comment on the fact I was 'a good son'. Whatever. I was glad to offer some pleasure, and the rhythm and silence and near body contact was pleasant to both of us.

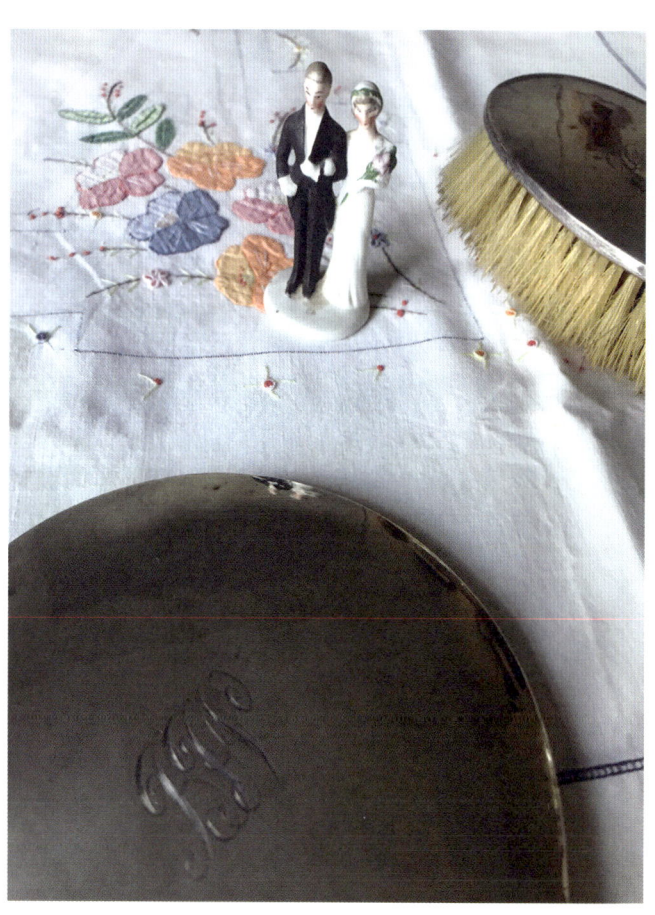

After Bess died I decided, very quickly, to keep the brush and mirror set. I realised it was pretty much worthless as an object, but the elegance of her monogram reminded me of a young woman who no longer existed, who had set out on life expecting certain things (which in fact were never delivered).

Today the mirror has some dents in it and seems rather small. As for the brush – it is one of my secret pleasures to pick it up and slowly brush my hair a few times with it. I smell my mother, I remember the hair-brushing, and my whole being relaxes completely. It's a short circuit of memory, complete to itself. Then I place the brush back on the shelf and I move on with my life.

This is my Christmas gift to you – Peace to all living and unseen creatures on earth.

December 27, 10.47 a.m.

I can still remember how embarrassed I was, as a kid, the way my mother felt perfectly at ease talking to strangers. It seemed conversation burst like birds from her mouth. It didn't matter if it was on the bus or in a veggie shop or just waiting at a crossing – she always had time for a few words, an exchange of views, a comment on the weather.

I on the other hand was shy, tongue tied and full of imaginings so vast I could not shape them with my tongue. It took me many years of writing and making films to try to empty these ideas and images out of my head. Even then they were obstinate and awkward-shaped, and it was only with true friends I felt at ease and could talk conversationally.

Yet recently, as I've said earlier, I have observed myself talking easily to anyone with time to listen. I can't think how this happened or rather when. Did it happen in hospital when time slowed right down and everything I'd fought to achieve suddenly seemed very small? Did my 'career' lose its stature beside the ordinary dramas of people trying to stay alive or achieve health? Perhaps.

I had slowed down too. After all, I literally could not move. I had time 'to pass the time of day', or the time of day would pass by me. But it was more than that. I understood for perhaps the first time that I was part of a huge world of humans all struggling to make sense of their situation, all of us equal, all of us struggling. I had stopped being a writer, etc – I was now just the patient in the bed in Room 13A. There is a curious equality there, implacable in its meaning.

I was suddenly interested in other people – I mean in what they had to say. Ordinary chat seemed to me not boring but actually a form of communication – was it like birds calling from tree to tree? Everything slowed down – right down. Just as it now takes me a long time to walk anywhere. For example this afternoon it took me a very long time and conscious effort to walk half a kilometre on crutches. I got tired and discouraged when I realised how far I had to go. The crutches bit into my armpits. I told myself to take it slowly, step by step. And it worked. But it was slow, almost agonising work.

So my whole relationship to time has altered. And I find myself chatting in shops, at bus stops, in just the way my mother once used to do. At the late age of 67 I have lost my shyness.

It makes me think of a sign I saw in an old English church: 'Stay, Gentle Passenger that Ye May Hear the Words of the

Deade'. It's not the latter part that interests me so much as the concept of us as 'gentle passengers' – all of us going somewhere together. We are carried into the future whether we want to or not. So we may as well chat as we travel forward into the future . . . Or remain silent, if that is preferred.

Yet for me this burst into chitchattery is very welcome and warming to the spirit. I think in the past I was actually frightened of people and what they thought of me. Now that thought never occurs to me. I am transparently what I am – an older man on crutches struggling along a very long road – and I say this without pity.

December 28, 6.55 a.m.

I awoke this morning filled with joy. Was it the absence of pain? The night before I had been out to a friend's place for dinner and ended up sitting uncomfortably. On the drive home I was in utter agony. Besides I had spent my time too ruthlessly all over the weekend, guzzling pleasures.

D and I had gone shopping. Shamelessly I spent a small fortune on a beautiful deep blue unlined jacket at my favourite menswear shop. We had gone here, there and everywhere, me on my crutches, running after pleasure as if chasing iridescent butterflies at dusk.

An old friend had come back from Britain and we lunched together, me pretending I was perfectly OK before I found the toilets were up an elaborately turned Victorian staircase which I aesthetically loved but which meant I could not use the toilets if I urgently needed to. (Returned to being an animal.)

The whole weekend had been a carnival of wants, of carelessness, of pretending I was okay now and like everyone else, except somehow I was on crutches (a skiing accident perhaps). D had been tender, careful, had cooked me beautiful meals full of invention. My oldest friend made a gorgeous peacock fan of a dinner party à trois and we sat round and laughed at time and circumstance.

Then I succumbed to the reality of pain on the way home and felt the small of my back was crumbling with each jerk of the tyres on the road. I was in agony.

Afterwards I drove myself hard into sleep, willing myself to lose consciousness – and strangely enough some kind god willed I did in fact lose consciousness. I did not wake up till 4.30 a.m., which for me is like waking up at 10.30 a.m. I lulled away time looking at FB messages, got up and made myself some herbal tea and toast, took it back to bed, then elided time away into a blissful rinse of sleep. So why did I awake at 6.55 a.m. filled with joy I cannot quite explain? Was it that I felt no pain? It was as if my body had magically melded itself together during the night, aided now by my own administration of pain relief, my own sense of how to adjust and change the settings. But it wasn't only this. As I looked out the window I could see the sun and the trees, everything so familiar that I felt so happy to be alive – even on these terms. I would get up and make D a coffee.

I enjoyed every aspect of this, being up early, looking out the window. And then I would make myself a cup of tea, I would slowly sink into another day, and all I felt was this sense of gratitude for being alive on a sunny Hawke's

Bay morning, with Parky the cat coming into my room and seeing me back in bed, jumping up on the rug, settling down with a shiver, and so we both began the adventure of another day – me improbably happy, my pain momentarily shelved, my dilemmas ignored or put aside for a while as I concentrated on the small change of living – the dollars and cents, coppers and pence without which we were told as children you could never make your fortune . . .

It is the small things that matter, the tiny courtesies in life. Of course the big questions loom too but let's put them in another basket for a while. Let's enjoy the sun . . .

The reality of why I am so happy. D and I have never enjoyed such intimacy as we do at present. We are closer than we ever have been, more simpatico. We spend a lot of time together, and just being together is heaven.

December 30, 1.13 p.m.

I'm preparing for the New Year – tidying my office. I have my chemotherapy which begins on 10 January and really stretches on through the foreseeable future – that is, May 2018. Because I have no idea how I'll respond I have to leave this area a blank, a no man's land. In my mind's eye I see it as a high bank of cloud which gradually occludes the light and settles all around me. Then it becomes a mist through which I am walking or wading. This goes on for quite a while, then the mist thins, then very slowly it lifts.

But realistically I have no idea what it will be like – except

I know it will be challengingly hard. I've lived these past few weeks as if chemo is never going to happen. I was going to say 'like a soldier who knows he is going off to war but lives as if the date of departure will never eventuate'. But all these similes and metaphors – mist, cloud, war – are inaccurate and that is what frightens me a little. I don't know what it will be like. It's the unknowable – though many people, including friends, have been through chemo and today are fully functioning people.

I have the cancer booklet which I have yet to sit down and read properly. I am like, 'Another day! Give me another day! Tomorrow and I'll start treating it seriously.' But realistically it is never going to happen, the reading, and that's the only way I can function at the moment.

Hence my tidying my office and preparing neat piles of papers of future projects. That is my form of optimism. That is my 'fuck you' to the fates, which I know is terribly dangerous – especially as I am pleading, at the same time, 'Only give me one more day . . .'

December 31

More memories.

It was a long time ago. Someone had the key to a bach on Waiheke, so we all crammed in together. It was that night I managed to sleep with him. Nobody took any notice because we were all young and that was being cool. It was the beginning of me falling in love. He was ready to fall in love too, and maybe that was it: we were both ready to be in love. Or was

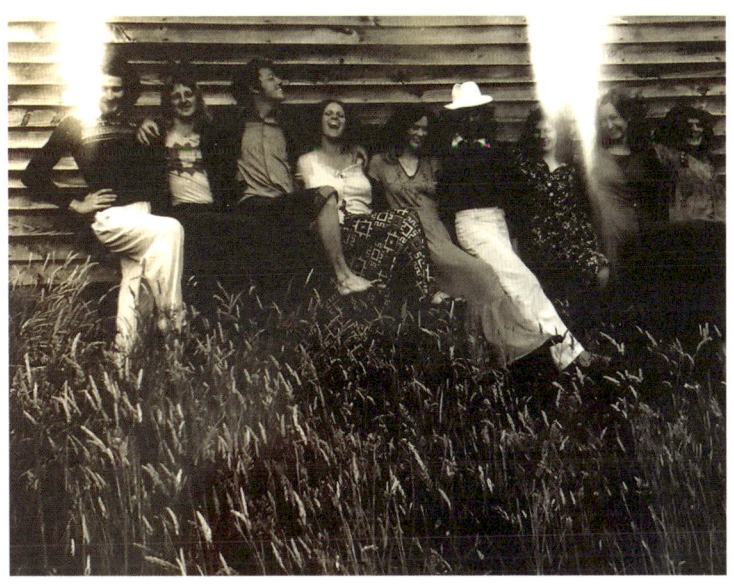

it a magical weekend? I was, in many ways, ill equipped for the enchantments and madness of a love affair. But that weekend, none of it mattered. All was lightness and ease.

Someone suggested we take a photograph. We went outside and almost naturally, in an excess of high spirits, we performed the drollery of a dance step. I managed to be right beside him. We were overwhelmed with the blithe spirit of happiness. Really we were strangers to one another. But in that moment all seemed possible.

Now, so many years later, he is dead and the boy beside us has committed suicide – and the love affair turned out to be a misfit which taught me a lot about myself. The photo seems to represent something else – it has a terseness the original moment lacked, a kind of bitter poetry, but there is still a beauty there, a lyricism I cannot help but see all over the surface of the photo, as much a part of it as that fault where the light leaked in and washed away the image, making it a one-off, an imperfect image. But for me, still, it evokes longing, the innocence of love, a moment in time in which I became myself and I experienced an almost impossible happiness.

January 2 2018, 4.41 a.m.

One of the interesting things with being sick is how people reveal themselves to you. Sometimes it's as if you are an abstract space which their actions (or non-actions) describe. For example: the old friend who sends his fervent best wishes but is never heard from again. You gather you are bad luck and somehow contagious, in the way that good luck is, like winning a lottery. The dear old friend who reportedly burst out weeping on hearing my news cannot ask me to my face about my 'illness'. (Is it an illness, a sickness? Is it a disease? What is it exactly except a fucking nuisance?) Or the acquaintance who becomes a friend simply by the act of listening very carefully and maintaining a discreet, watchful silence as if picking up clues (like how can I help you?).

Generally 'Let me know if there is any way I can help you – any way –' means I'll never hear from you again. Sickness is embarrassing, sickness is dirty. It's true too. I have much less control over my bodily fluids now but I also feel less fear about this, less mortal embarrassment.

It is not that I have lost shame but I have become more at home with the inconveniences of having a body which will not perform its habitual duties. I live with my body much more intimately now. I listen to it. Once upon a time my body was its own ruthless machine, demanding pleasure. My body was like a cruel master and my mind was a very distant duenna, like a landlord who has lost control of his tenant's actions. Now I live with my body all through the long hours of the night and during the equally long hours of the day. You could say my body and I are trapped together on this adventure.

But back to the way people react. Some people, completely unasked, are kind. For example a woman bakes me a banana loaf and delivers it quietly and without expectation of conversation or applause. Then there is the old friend, the one who knows me best, who has been away in another city so has not seen me at all. He comes and visits, then he talks about himself exuberantly, his ills and pains, his latest problem with his career, his future plans. I await the space for him to ask about me, my situation – what it was like finding myself in hospital, for example? This never happens. A forlorn feeling overtakes me but I maintain face. Eventually he leaves, registering surprise that I need crutches to see him off at the door. Is he embarrassed by my neediness? By my fall from grace?

I struggle myself with my own attitude to what's happened to me, and have to learn to accommodate myself to the disease's dictates, so I guess I should cut some slack to my friends and acquaintances. The chemo booklet which I quickly read yesterday afternoon, on New Year's Day, is pretty explicit about what lies ahead. The way I feel today may be the best I'll feel for quite a while. So I guess what I am saying is, I'm as little in control of what is happening to me as my friends are in control of their reactions.

I cut them some slack because I know I and my body are in it for the long haul. It's not quick, whatever is happening to me, so I should be generous and accept that reactions to me, to it, to the situation, will be various – and probably they will change over time. But some part of me is observant, as observant of others as I am of myself. I am – for better or for worse – ruthlessly observant.

This is not necessarily a kind virtue. In fact, it may not possess virtue at all. It is like a compulsion, something to do with the lack of time – an impatience with what is involved in pretence. At the same time this doesn't mean I know what I'm doing. I need to learn the art of kindness. I need to be humble and kind. That pretty much means I am neither. I am irascible, impatient and irritated by what has happened to me. I guess I need to accept that other people, even old friends, will have attitudes which are all over the place too. It's not like it's uncharted territory so much as a constantly changing one – including my own attitude to what's happening to me. I apologise for writing this so soon after New Year's Day when everyone is feeling so . . . up?

January 4, 3.43 a.m.

As if it's not bad enough having cancer, my right foot has recently swollen in size. This is depressing. I tried to tell myself I had been overdoing the walking (albeit with Freddie, the walker) so the swelling was just a result of overuse. But my doctor (in Auckland) said it might be deep vein thrombosis. O joy. So I went to a 24/7 doctor yesterday (in Napier) who gave me a blood test form but said, however, he thought it was a complication from tinea. I had to come back to the 24/7 doctor to get the results today. This ended up being a two-and-a-quarter-hour wait in which there appeared to be no doctor, though the odd accident victim emerged triumphantly bandaged up. Eventually I saw a doctor who gave me a form for a scan tomorrow. It was perfectly timed so the scanning place was closed. So I have another day of waiting.

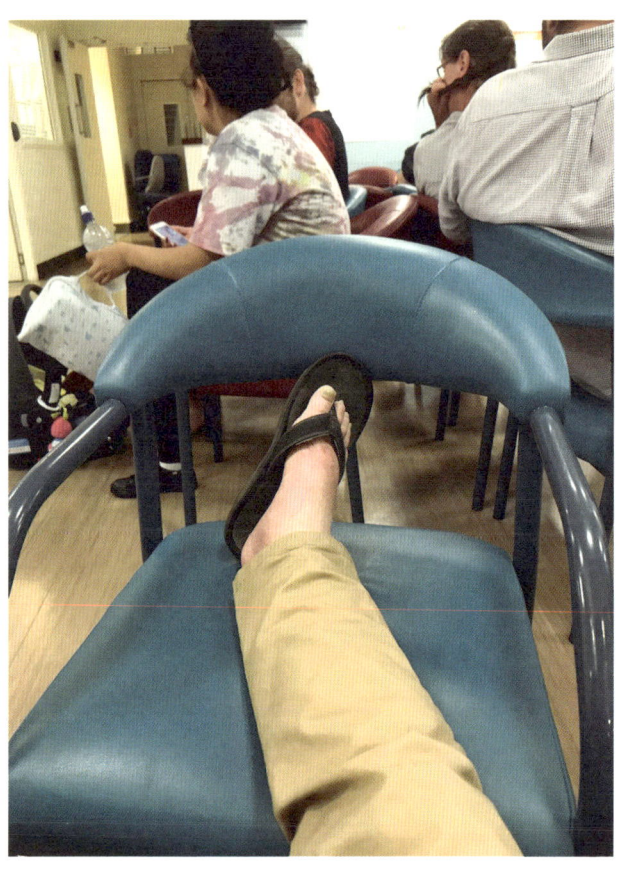

January 5, 2.44 p.m.

I do not have a clot. Wonderful news. I also have 'very photographic veins', according to the pleasant young woman who
did the screening. I'm thrilled.

January 7, 4.34 a.m.

I have a lot of time on my hands and I decided to look back.

1.

There is the thing where you say you remember something but
really you remember the photo itself. This is a case in point.
I'm nine in this small square Box Brownie photo (page 106).
The photo itself is the size of a large postage stamp. I am
formally posed beside a wooden tub holding a pine tree. But it
is the self-selected formality of my pose which strikes me now.
I seem to be very composed inside myself – almost secretive to
myself. But note the scarf drawn up so tightly to the toggle, plus
the socks beautifully pulled up. In another period I might have
made a Hitler Youth. I'm also a kind of eternal virgin – not in
a sexual sense since my sense of sexuality is only nascent and
primitive at this stage – but I am made to be fodder to older
boys who will enjoy pulling down my long socks (what does
that signify?) and loosening that stranglehold of a scarf. I'm a
believer in all the arcane late-imperial African codes of Boy
Scouting or its junior equivalent 'Cubbing'. The expectation
is I will become a Scout (I didn't – trouble ahead – officially

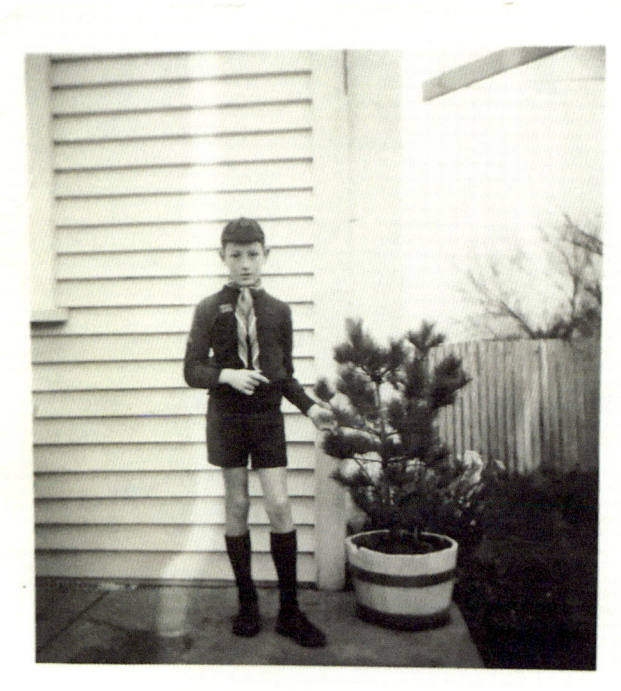

because I couldn't manage the dictionary of knots, but realistically I retired confused before the onslaught of incipient male sexuality and general rowdiness).

I would have made a good nun. This little photo could have served as my certificate.

It's my body language that so interests me here. Who told me to pose with some of the stillness and eloquence of a medieval painting, with my finger pointing significantly to the tree? My legs seem placed just so as well. And why point to the tree? It had a life in our family, coming back as a seedling from Lake Rotoma where we occasionally holidayed in a motor camp. In a way it is an aide memoire to holiday times, to good times, to something special. It was placed in the wooden tub which the last house owner had left behind. This meant it could be shifted inside as a Christmas tree until its robust growth meant that Dad officially ended its life. It had outgrown its suburban need, so it was destroyed. To me the tree has some kind of animus, is an unspeaking person. The fact it used to be decorated with tinsel and crepe paper, with presents nestling at its feet, indicated it was somehow a magic tree – a giving tree.

Maybe that's why I seem to be secretly pointing to it in a gesture which says 'the tree, not me'. I'm already perfecting the art of deflection. But it's the perfection of my performance which is heart-breaking in this tiny square of remembrance. It all means so much: the perfect Cub uniform, the shoes and socks and, even worse, the cap pulled on so tightly to my skull. Then there's my other hand, as in an advertisement, lightly touching the pine needles as if to further illustrate my point (the tree, not me).

But there is some other 'grammar' inside this photo which points to the way this little manikin is held in a confining present. First of all there is the dreary black-and-whiteness of it, symbolic of the limited choices of the period. There is no colour. It's all a pervasive grey. Then there are the strong lines of horizontals – weatherboards, then the verticals – the wooden fence in the background, the clothesline that can just be seen at the top. It's like I'm captured inside a parallelogram of lines. That's the grid I'm growing up amidst or even against. As Joan Didion says, that's how I 'participated in the paranoia' of my time.

Revolt, unhappiness, change of direction: this will all come. The pine tree will be yanked out of the tub, killed off, then burnt in the back yard with that special smell of burning pine needles. I won't attend the pyre, as already I will be growing up into my own confusions about who and what I am and where the fuck on earth do I possibly fit in?

This photo is all about the terror and conformity of being 'a good boy', which was my conception of myself then. I had no idea how this would almost destroy me. At this time, however, it seems to fit me like a seamless glove.

Can I remember the photo being taken? I don't think so. Yet looking into this photograph I recognise a self which causes me a certain degree of grief amid the hilarity: is it possible to see a self which is so lacking in knowledge about what life will deliver that it is almost shocking?

2.

Every so often an amateur photographer manages to take a photo that takes on all the aspects of a classic photograph. You see it often with snaps – some rare moment is caught on film, underlining the element of chance inherent to all photography. Roland Barthes talked of punctum, 'that accident

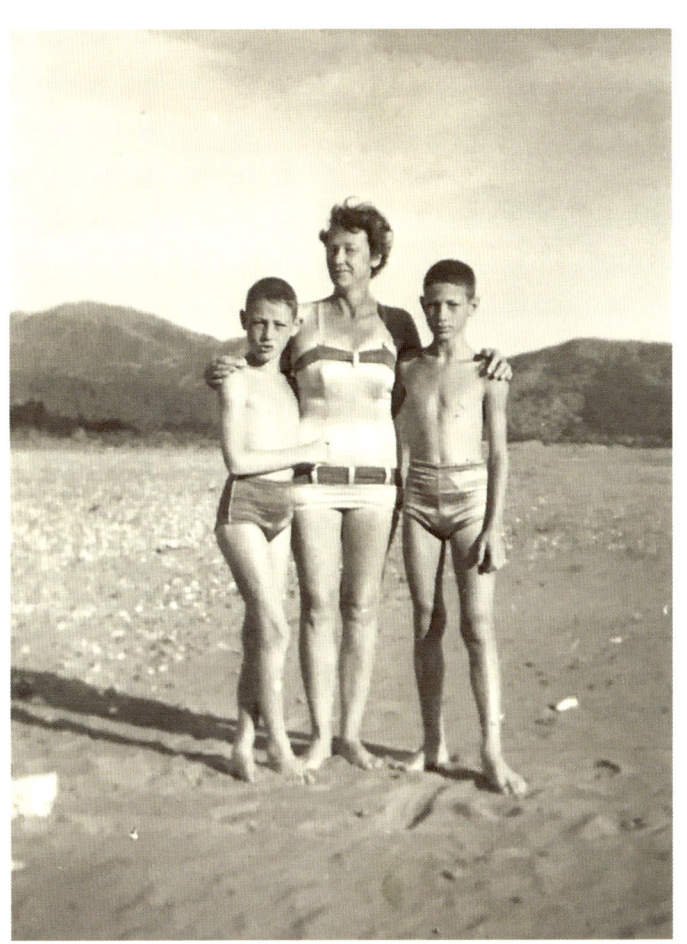

which pricks, bruises me', meaning an element in a photograph that causes you to become momentarily, almost internally, still. This photo has punctum.

It was taken by my father, Gordon, on a holiday we had in 1959–1960 around the East Cape. The beach is Hicks Bay/ Wharekahika and it was a paradisial holiday. All families, be they ever so remotely functional, usually select one holiday place as the ultimate one they ever enjoyed. This was ours.

But there are one or two things about the photograph that I want to comment on. One is that Dad is standing a long way back. We are isolated within the frame by landscape which is as much a character in the photo as we are – the stretch of sand with its bank of shells, the abandoned towels (actually towels and a piece of canvas from Dad's experience of sand in the Desert War), the distant hills and the overarching sky. There is a distant lip of sea. We are enclosed in the landscape, yet isolated within it, formally arranged, unsmiling. I cannot say what urged my father to pick up the camera and take a photograph that says, 'Here, this is my family. Let all the world see.'

Also, why was Dad standing so far back? What stopped him taking five steps forward so we came into more informal contact, which might have led to a smiling, joking photo. Or did that possibility not exist either?

In those economical days you did not waste film, so there is only one shot. That makes the grace of the photo all the more outstanding. Another interesting thing: my mother Bess did not suggest that she take a photo of Dad with us. There is no photo of Dad guarding his sons on this epochal holiday. It was like that language did not exist.

Some further things about this photograph. I seem to have

naturally taken on the same supine body language as in the Cub photograph. I'm aged nine, slightly older than the Cub photo. I'm inclined into my mother's body, fitting neatly into the curve of her hip and breast, my shoulder fitting under her arm pit. We're two parts of a jigsaw that fit. I seem to be speaking and she seems to be listening. My mother, quite naturally – without any consciousness of European art and the iconic status of Mary and Jesus – widens her arms to encompass and embrace her sons. My brother Russell, two years older, stands up straighter than me, staring intently, even moodily into the camera. If this were another kind of painting he would hold a holster and a sheath of arrows. He is a young princeling, aged eleven. I keep reaching for classical analogies for this very simple snap that occurred as an act of magic on an East Coast beach – a synergy which allowed the inner form of the family to take visual form, even down to my father's distanced yet accurate viewpoint down the viewfinder. (It was a knock-off Rolleiflex camera where you looked down into a beautiful glassy slightly convex sheet. It was with this camera that I first began image-making.) Interestingly, given the late period, the photo is still in black and white rather than gaudy colour (an economy measure: my mother would have regarded casual family photos as very low down on the list of 'what was important').

This photo quickly became representative of my family. It was used as the cover on my memoir *Long Loop Home*, though slightly skewered. It is also inside the cover of *Dear Oliver* in a cropped version. Probably there is no photo which better expresses the economy of our family life but also, almost accidentally, its beauty and impossibility.

I have no memory of the photo being taken.

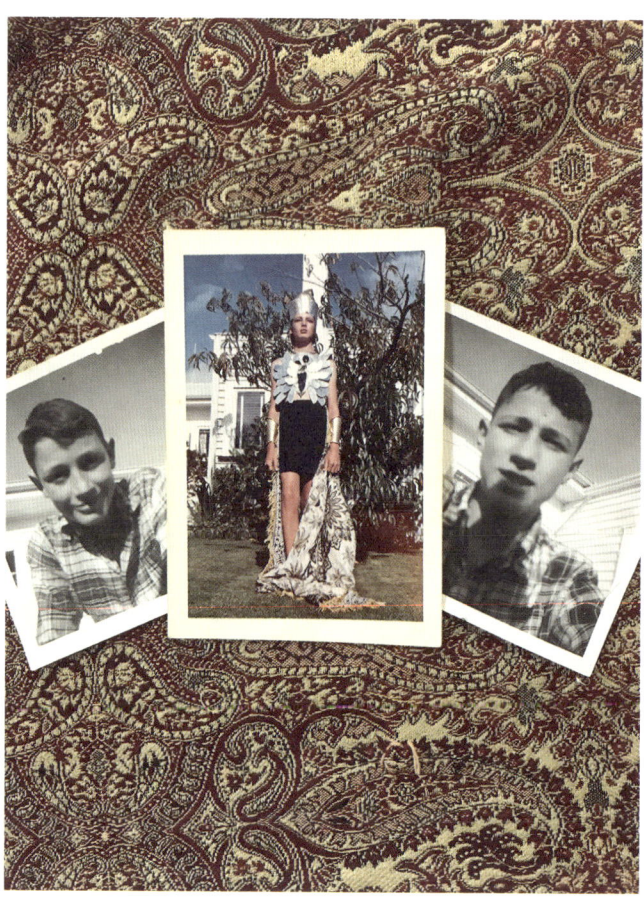

3.

I am 12 in this photographic montage. It is 1962. Two years before, an 'uncle' invited himself into my life. I was never the same afterwards. But like many people in this situation, I lived in a compartmentalised way. There was that, and I never knew what 'that' was – it was blank and ominous. And then there was the rest of my life. None of it made sense. I could not match the two parts up, so I just lived with them, ill-fitting and jagged.

Pasadena Intermediate each year had a costume ball. Russell, to the right, made me this extraordinary costume to wear. It was the product of his obsessiveness. I could not conceptualise that he was in love with me but I could feel the heat of his obsession. This led to a strange push–pull in our relationship, an unreality and a peculiar form of denial and pursuit. I would not say he idolised me, as he didn't. But perhaps you could say he fetish-ised me. Some already damaged part of me played up to it. I was both more adult than my years and completely retarded: stuck back at the age of eleven when the 'uncle' emerged in my life. As you can see, this was a complicated period of trying to negotiate difficult emotional currents which didn't necessarily make sense.

The film *Cleopatra* had recently come out, so there was a vogue for all things Hollywood-Egyptian. But the costume also pays homage to Yul Brynner in *The Ten Commandments*: he was an exceptionally sexy King of Egypt to Charlton Heston's equally sexy Moses. The costume is what today you would call 'gender fluid'. Russell and I were both gay, of course, though in saying this you immediately get into a thicket of semantics. Also – at what point does consciousness alight on self-realisation? To both of us it was 'just' a costume. Ostensibly.

I do find it very hard to say anything further about this photo except it allowed me to wear what was basically a miniskirt, heavy eye make-up and lipstick in public at the age of 12. As you can see, I wore it with a lot of attitude. At the same time I am not sure (I no longer know that boy) I wanted to wear make-up, lipstick and a miniskirt. (I can remember the waxy thickness of lipstick on my lips and how I hated it. Lipstick stolen from our mother.) But as an act of outrage it thrilled me.

This photo was undoubtedly taken by my brother wanting to archive his masterpiece. This was done when Dad was at golf on Sunday, as he disliked intensely what appeared to be my feminisation. It was a bold statement, that costume. So bold that I cannot recall what the reaction was. I think I may have been in some sort of trance when I wore it to the ball – I was Cleopatra, the King of Egypt, the Queen of Sheba. But this is interesting: I had a 'girlfriend' and I hoped it impressed her. We were 'in love with one another' and sent each other love notes. I do recall after the costume ball Valerie's father said she should stay away from me. This was so hard to understand. I remember trying to understand it but failing to. He could see something in me I couldn't see in myself. My most vivid memory is that the headpiece did not fit and rubbed against the back of my neck: the whole contrivance of the costume, as the evening went on, was increasingly annoying.

So the local details stayed with me while I missed out on the big picture. But what was the big picture exactly? What were we unconsciously saying to our local community? We couldn't come out, my brother and me, as coming out as an act did not philosophically exist in 1963. Besides, neither of us was conscious of what that meant – to be gay. We were not conscious of anything more than the pleasure of producing an

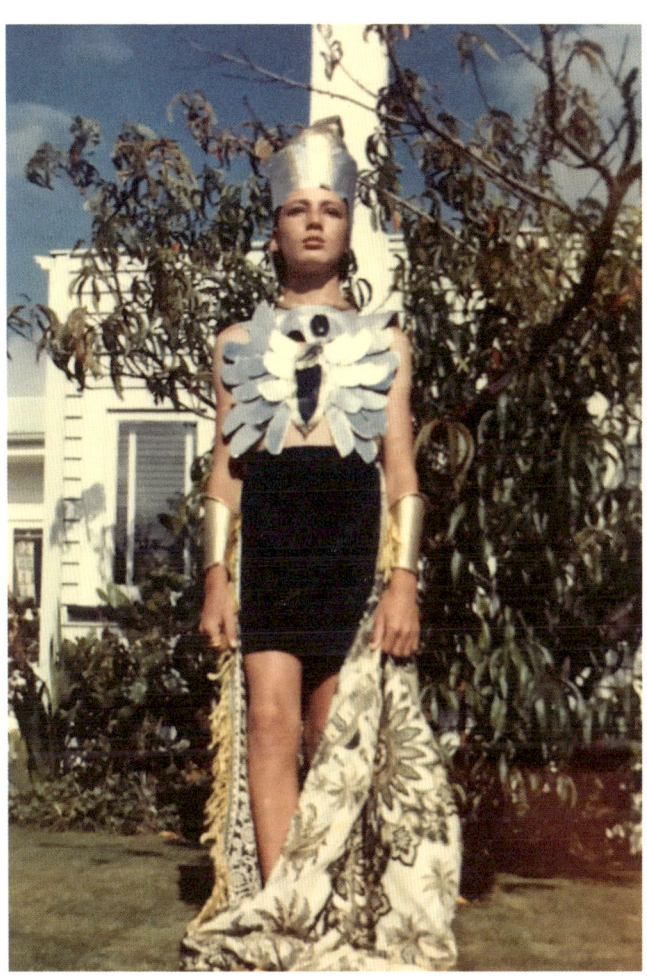

outrage. We wanted to say something but we didn't know what it was.

I no longer have access to the mind of that boy. He is so far away from me as to be unknown. But I understand it was, in its own small way, an act of rebellion. And I was happy to take part.

4.

In 1968 – five years after the Cleopatra costume – I was unlucky enough to 'win the ballot' by which young New Zealand men were offered the opportunity to go to fight in Vietnam. I was 18. First of all you had to undergo a medical test. This was done in Fort Cautley in Devonport. I went there with the other young men, all of whom were understandably nervous. I was determined not to go to Vietnam. I was deeply opposed to the war, but also I knew I would not survive such a brutally masculinist society. I had decided to say I was homosexual. This was in advance of my actually accepting I was gay. It's a very hard thing to explain, how the human mind operates, especially the mind of an 18-year-old who, to a degree, had been through a childhood sexual trauma.

When I got into the doctor's room, I announced that I was homosexual. At this point the doctor's foot slammed the door shut. But I had something bigger on my mind. I would not undress. By this age, I was phobic about my body, which I was convinced was so ugly other humans could not look at it without feeling sick (it was a kind of body dysmorphia), but I also felt I would get an uncontrollable erection if another male so much as looked at me. This neatly represented the dichotomy of my position. I was fucked. Or, more to the point, I was locked, as a machine seizes up when trying to go in two different directions at once. The long ago 'uncle' episode had frozen me with fear and I felt disgusting and ugly. This was a crushing reality to me. But almost separate from this and having nothing to do with it, I was also a randy young teenager overwhelmed by the erotic power of boys and men. I could not work out how to resolve the contradictions of my situation.

There were two doctors, one old school, the other the kind of doctor who appeared in the serials of women's magazines – I immediately fell in love with him. Meanwhile I was aware I was in a very dangerous situation. The old-school doctor said I could go to prison for refusing to obey orders (to strip).

I was staunch. I stood there and said I didn't care. I was not undressing. I was gay. That invalidated me for military service. This astonishes me now. I was a shy boy, almost crippled with fear about speaking to strangers.

But in this situation I had no hesitation about how I would act. The old-school doctor immediately jumped up and started a sort of phobic washing of his hands. I was filth? He was Herod?

The young doctor persuaded him I was serious, that they had to accept my statement.

I felt victorious. But this was not the end of the incident. It was the army, after all, and there was an almost stereotypically sadistic sergeant who kept us all waiting till the doctors left. He then insisted, quite against regulations, on looking at all our papers (on which the doctors had written whatever comments they needed to make). This was in a room in which all we boys sat petrified. We were so very young. When he got to mine, he made an expressive sound of disgust, and let the paper fall from his fingers as if the mere touch of paper was defiling. The paper flew down to the floor. In a fit of utter anger, I scooped it up. He had stigmatised me. But he had done something else too. He had confirmed something within myself that I barely understood. I was stronger than I thought. I could speak up when it counted. This was a victory.

At the same time I still occupied the shell of this conflicted boy or young man. Yes, I had said, at the point of a gun so to speak, I was homosexual. But – and this is how extraordinary human nature is – I quickly resolved that this was an expediency that did not relate to any personal truth or reality. In other words, I walked out of that military establishment no more accepting I was gay than when I went in. I could not yet afford to be free.

Interestingly for this year I cannot find a photograph of myself. Make of that what you will.

5.

This is me at 22. It's 1972. It's four years after being called up for the Vietnam medical. Without my knowing it I'm about to leave one part of my life as efficiently as exiting a building and never being seen again. My face is tranquil and unformed as soft wax. I'm rocking a kind of 1905 Russian revolutionary period look, mixed with a James Taylor wandering-down-a-country-road vibe. I'm wearing a poloneck pullover, inevitably green to contrast with my auburn hair. And look at all that hair, handfuls of it. I have a tiny little rather unconvincing Marxist moustache and beard. I'm heterosexual in the photo, or trying to be. It's my last impression.

It's a youth hostel card and I used it as I travelled down the South Island, heading for Dunedin where I aimed to find a flat and start writing a D.H. Lawrence-like novel. I saw myself as a writer, though there was no evidence for it, apart from my

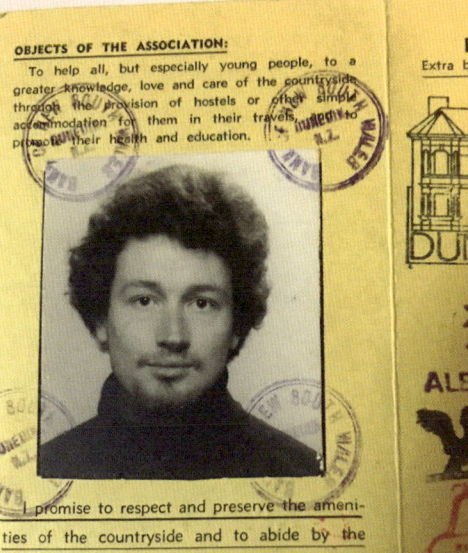

I promise to respect and preserve the amenities of the countryside and to abide by the Rules and Regulations for the use of Youth Hostels.

Signature ....

Occupation ....student.............

HOSTELS

Extra blanks obtainable fr

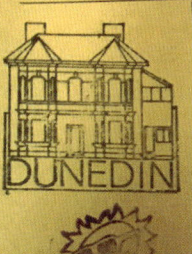

DUNEDIN

ALEXANDRA

shag point

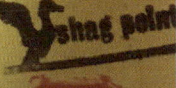

This Card is valid
Youth Hostel in th
arrangements have be

diaries and all my unpublished writing – and my burning desire to become a writer. Yet as a person I was an unrealised human with an enormous amount of conflict behind me – and within me (the making of a writer?). How the two were to come together – unrealised being/work of art – I do not know. (I did not publish a book until I was 41.)

In referring to the photo of me as a Cub I talked briefly about the terror and conformity of being a good boy. Simone de Beauvoir wrote about the horror of being a young bourgeoise and how the expectations of good/'refined' behaviour were so claustrophobic they eventually led to her revolt against not only her very powerful mother but also society. I too had a powerful mother and I tried for a long time to live up to her expectations that I be a heterosexual grammar school boy – an unconvincing portrayal on my part, I'm afraid.

But I'm in the last vestiges of trying to be a good boy in this photo. This meant, primarily, denying the fact I was gay. Oh god, how much time I wasted on this pretence. I wanted to please my parents. I didn't know who I was. Or else, and this is infinitely possible, it was my excuse for 'having a girlfriend'.

This is something that fills me with shame still: that I had a love affair with a young woman who had no idea I was homosexual. This pretence went on for at least 18 months. We lived together in Dunedin but it was a *mariage blanc*. I wasted her life. It can have only made her doubt herself. I was a shit – a terminally confused shit who didn't know himself.

I can see looking back there was a whole lot of stuff that sent me uncontrollably out of the gate trying to be heterosexual. That 'uncle' who molested me made me want to be straight. It seemed a way of denying any contact, any contamination. Besides, heterosexuality was what my parents wanted and what child does not want to please her or his parents? Yet how feeble this sounds. How very feeble. There's a lot of waste and damage on the way to growing up, to being mature. So this photo, which looks so peaceful and in which I look so placid, is in fact the face of a pretender, the mask of a man pretending to be someone other than himself. But it's also the face of someone who had reached the end of the road. That road. I would abruptly change course here. I would accept my homosexuality.

I look at this photo in a different way to the way I looked at myself as a nine-year-old Cub. I don't – for whatever reason – grant myself the pity I grant to him. Is it that I am more of an accomplice? Do you become the accomplice in your own life as you grow older? I would say yes. Generally speaking I would say I am pretty hard on myself – I can still hear my parents' condemning voices in my head, and in some way I can never be right or do right, no matter what I do or achieve. (My parents as they got old, however, granted me their approval.) But forgive myself? That's much harder.

This has been a difficult piece for me to write. I hate exposing the fact that I lived with a young woman, that I was a fake. (Though I recognise it is virtually a gay rite of passage.) I lay awake in bed last night fretting about how I would write this and even whether I should post it. But anyway here it is – a photo of me as a closeted young man just on the point I was about to open the closet door.

'I tore myself away from the safe comfort of certainties through my love for truth – and truth rewarded me.'
– Simone de Beauvoir

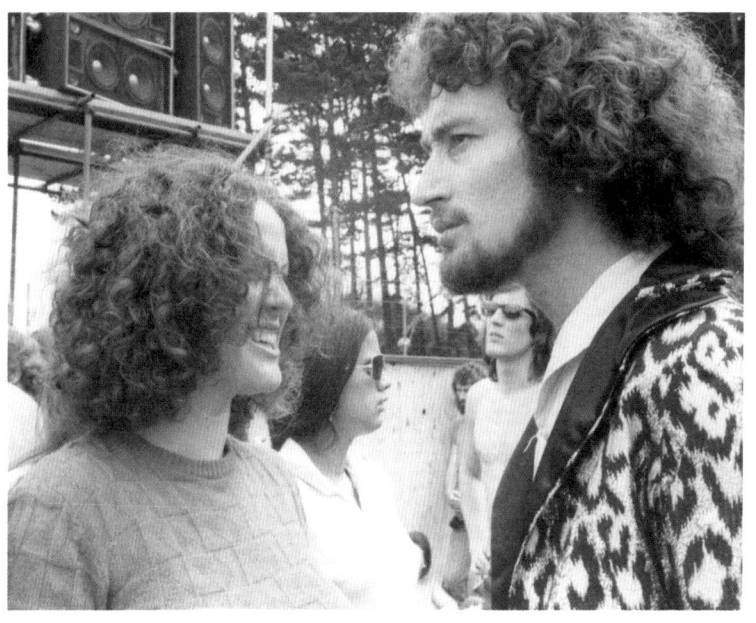

6.

This is me at the Rolling Stones concert in Western Springs. Bear in mind this is one year after the youth hostel photo. I was running wild, running free. I had taken acid. I had fallen in love. I had found friends. Friends like me. The music in our ears was Roxy Music, David Bowie, the Stones at their most flamboyant and lascivious (Mick's outfit was a revealing sky-blue body stocking stitched all over with little gold mirrors). It was the time of 'the low spark of high heeled boys', as the song goes. Of boys wearing make-up. Of 'walking on the wild side'. I had arrived at a peak moment of gender fluidity: I had come out at the most perfect time. Whatever was latent in the Cleopatra costume revealed itself now as having been a harbinger of things to come. I enjoyed the oxygen of outrage. Gay Liberation emerged. I joined up. Everything about my life expanded just as the traumas of my past contracted, shrivelled, seemed to vanish to a distant point no bigger than a freckle. It was a time of parties and forgetting. Those other grieving secret selves were buried (and forgotten). In fact I disclaimed them, any ownership of them.

I made up a past and instantly became it. I was unaware the past cannot be dismissed so lightly, so blithely. It lies inside each one of us, waiting to pounce. But at that moment I felt only the freedom of no longer carrying its huge weight. (I failed to understand that most of my contemporaries also carried burdens from the past.) I thought I could walk free. It was glorious, and I will always remember this period as the happiest of my life, the moment I became myself.

I would be more or less the same continuous character from now on for the rest of my life.

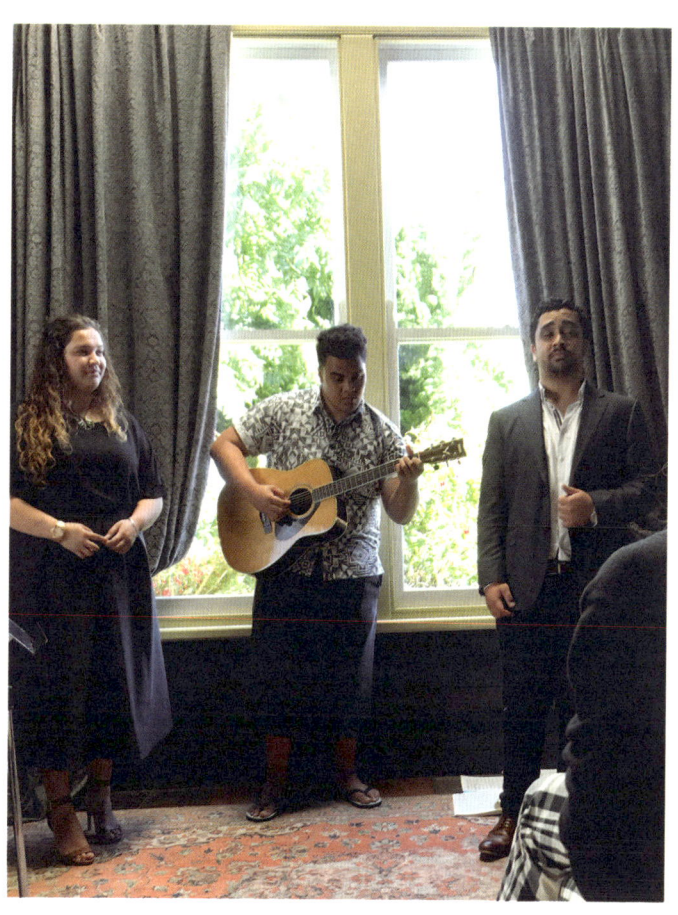

I've never been very good when I'm given something. I tend to freeze up and become completely artificial just when I should be most genuine. I can't work out quite why this is. The fact is I'm genuinely moved by the smallest gift. But it's best to catch me off guard.

Sometimes I've wondered if I don't feel worthy of such gifts. This gets a little closer to the truth. There's a whole pool of unworthiness in most of us, a compound of childhood inferiority, maybe not bring praised enough. I'm old enough to come from the generation whose parents never praised or even commented on our progress or excellence or lack thereof. They may have felt things but it was never verbalised. When I was a sprinter, for example, Dad who'd been a sprinter himself, never came to watch me run. Did this make me hungry for compliments? Thirsty for approval? You bet.

But this is all leading up to a beautiful event that was so far away from my expectations I was reduced, in a way, to being a spellbound little boy at my first circus or play – which I can remember vividly as two of the key events of my life. (It was when I came awake. It was how I discovered the world of art, and artifice.)

This is what happened. Anna Pierard had been following my Facebook postings and got in touch and offered to put on some music at D's and my house here in Napier. This seemed thrilling, but I had no real idea of how it would go or what it would mean.

This is what it meant. Think of the studio in all its dusky late-afternoon glory, chairs arranged facing the windows with their heavy theatrical drapes, so in effect it becomes a stage. Outside the windows, the blaze of the garden. (Think colonial-Visconti, if such a thing were possible – an elegant room awaiting an audience.)

Anna brought along her mother Jane and, as a special guest, Madeleine Pierard. I had last seen her in an astonishing, blow-you-away performance of *Nixon in China* at Auckland's Town Hall. And here she was in my house, in the studio in Napier . . . But it wasn't only this family ensemble, which lent its own intimate charm. Anna had brought along three students from Project Prima Volta. (This is a project which develops young singers in Hawke's Bay, professionalises them, tunes them up for the 21st century and reveals their talent and, by way of the same process, burnishes their self-esteem and reveals to them a whole world of options they may not have thought of.) Anna is to be praised to the heavens for this entirely worthy project. There are a lot of rootless kids left in the dust of Hawke's Bay, their souls withering and dying.

This evening she brought along Catherine in killer heels; Emmanuel dressed in a lavalava and huge black beads, a gentle giant of a man; and the smaller-statured Taylor.

First, we had the two Pierard sisters singing duets from Mozart. There is nothing like two women singing in harmony, their voices rising and rising ever higher. Make that two sisters, and the dynamic becomes more fascinating. I sat there mute. Beauty was everywhere, was actual, existed in that room as we all sat there exulting in the gift of sound – of music. We relaxed, bathed, immersed ourselves in the glory of it.

The final part of the programme was 'the young people' who took command of the stage superbly and won our hearts with their simplicity, engagement and – yes, talent. Each of them sang beautifully. Taylor sang in Italian. Emmanuel charmed with his big heart and big voice. The final performance was Katherine singing 'La vie en rose' which she did in the way water flecks out from a fountain filled with joy, melancholy, a rush of feeling. I wept. Rose sitting beside me wept.

I forgot – I forgot the fact I start chemotherapy in a few days. Wasn't this the greatest of gifts?

When the young people sang I saw, too, how nurturing sweetens the soul. They have been coached, encouraged, brought towards the light, given something to aspire to. They rewarded us with performances that enriched us in turn. How far away from self-neglect, or the knife of self-hatred buried deep in the heart, the curdled self which so many of us grew up with.

Later we had Prosecco and superb food cooked by a dear friend, Annie Gascoigne. What richnesses were heaped here, what joy, what beauty speckled the heavens for a few brief hours.

Back in fucking hospital. Excuse my French. I could cry with rage. Weep with self-pity. It's my foot. The oncologist wants me to be blasted intravenously with antibiotics before I can reach chemotherapy, which now seems some Immaculate Portal I can only ever strive to enter.

I'm sitting in Triage at Auckland Hospital awaiting direction. Offscreen I can hear a tubercular, hacking cough. I'm not even good enough to have chemo, it seems. Healthy enough. I have to have my ghastly foot or feet salved of tinea so I can enter chemotherapy in a virgin state of skin-innocence.

D took the wrong turning to Emergency as he drove me here (chronically bad signposting at the hospital – hate to be in a real emergency round here). And while D was backing out of a dead end I spotted the 'Temporary Mortuary'. I thought to myself, 'Why don't you just drop me off here. It would save a lot of trouble. I'm bound for there sooner or later, why not cut to the chase?'

Pardon my raw emotions. I just didn't think it'd be a 'return to go' so quickly. Welcome to the life of a semi-demi-forever invalid.

Then it suddenly strikes me: this is admissions in Emergency, as in *ER*, as in every other medical television programme. Why isn't it so dramatic? Not that I want dramatic. In fact I don't want to be here at all.

Now it's later and I'm in an intermediate admission zone. I'm back in the hell of the yellow and black curtains.

Next door to me is a silent guy who's just been told they want to enter his body through his penis. The smooth doctor has outlined the possible problems – blood-contamination,

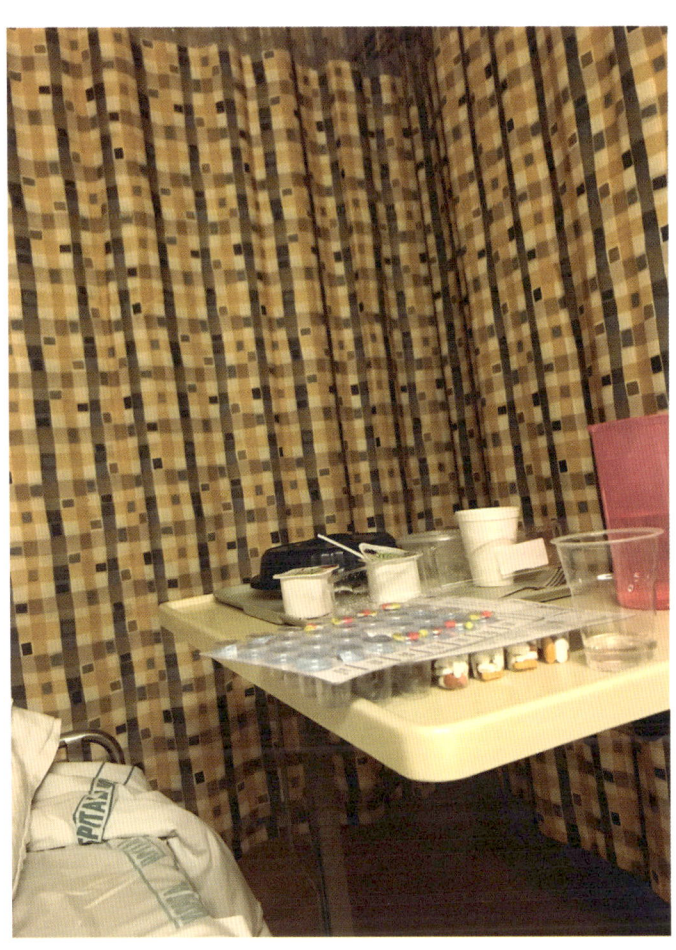

HIV – each of them percussively ending with an OK? The guy next door is totally silent.

The fact is I guess I'm lucky to be here being looked after. Though the young doctor before asked me if I was 'confused'. This was followed by questions about the year, who was prime minister, her name – standard Alzheimer's questions. Charming. I thought I was in here for a bung foot.

January 11, 5.18 a.m.

I didn't understand that was how it would be. Bits would fail. I didn't comprehend that was how it would happen. Or least of all – so quickly. It gives me some idea of my shortened life span – that parts would start failing so soon. I had seen myself as robust and capable of withstanding knocks. But this fat foot episode has revealed to me how vulnerable I am.

I spend a demoralising 24 hours at the lowest level of hospital care, wherein it's hard to get the attention of a nurse. I'm left to stew in my impotence once I know I'm going home, but there's no one to sign it off, no one to even ask. You're just left there in a hospital bed you don't want to be in, desperate to get away but unable to effect even the simplest thing: departure.

Once I was released I had the mild euphoria of a hostage set free. On the bus home I couldn't stop looking – and marvelling – at clouds, crowds of people going about their business, the random beauty of people not confined to a bed. Everything seemed rich and textured and full of an amazing energy. Once home I felt blessed to be within a house with rooms, with Ajax ready to roll over and greet me with the expanse – as big as a polar cap – of his white furry tummy. I'm alive, I think to myself: I'm not dead yet, I'm OK – for the time being.

I suddenly realised that this is how it might play out – small secondary problems/failures which bit by bit drag me down. I was so upset I forgot to have my evening pills and I awoke this morning creaky with pain. (I had also forgotten to have my incredibly important pre-chemo blood test.) My fat foot had obsessed me, upset me. I lost my bearings. Almost completely.

I had spent too long on FB, I lost my bearings in relation to reality, obligations. I was lost. That is what I was. Lost.

Later:
The oncology clinic says I can be booked into the Monday chemo session. Rather than something to fear, this now appears almost a triumph. I know my vulnerability now. I know small secondary infections can bring me down. There's nothing grand about it. It's obscure, belittling, deeply human – ordinary. I have to regard everything as 'important' – every swelling, mark on my gums, ache.

January 12, 4.01 a.m.

I can't write anything at present.

January 15, 4.49 a.m.

The relationship of human to animal is a complex one. Shorten the gaze to human and animal companion, and it becomes even more fraught with emotion. I'm writing this in the aftermath of my much-loved cat Parky being run over four days ago, while I was up in Auckland not getting chemo last week.

Let me explain. Parky is a small black and white female cat which D and I have owned for seven or eight years. She is – was – an intimate, charming, wilfully obstinate little animal. She had already almost died when she was struck by a car crossing the road. She disliked being approached frontally and it was only by a set of stratagems that I managed to actually get hold of her and caress her. Her eyes were always wild, yet you could have set a watch by her regularity. She always appeared in the evening, jumping up on a red blanket at the end of our bed, which she approached dramatically, as a high jumper might a particularly high hurdle. Her fur was thick and often bedazzled with mist. She would then sit down and curate her fur for a seemingly endless amount of time. But after this she would settle down, and in proximity and even intimacy she would roll over and present her stomach. At the same time she was ready to award you with a swipe for over-familiarity.

Timid, wild, beautiful, individual – she was all of those things. She did not appear yesterday, and today, after I put notices in the neighbours' letterboxes about a lost cat, a neighbour rang and said they had found a dead cat on their front lawn. It looked like the photo I had put up of Parky.

Parky, beautiful, alive and wild, was now dead.

I apologise for rhapsodising over the death of a mere moggy, but Parky was part of my defence. She was a stout wall

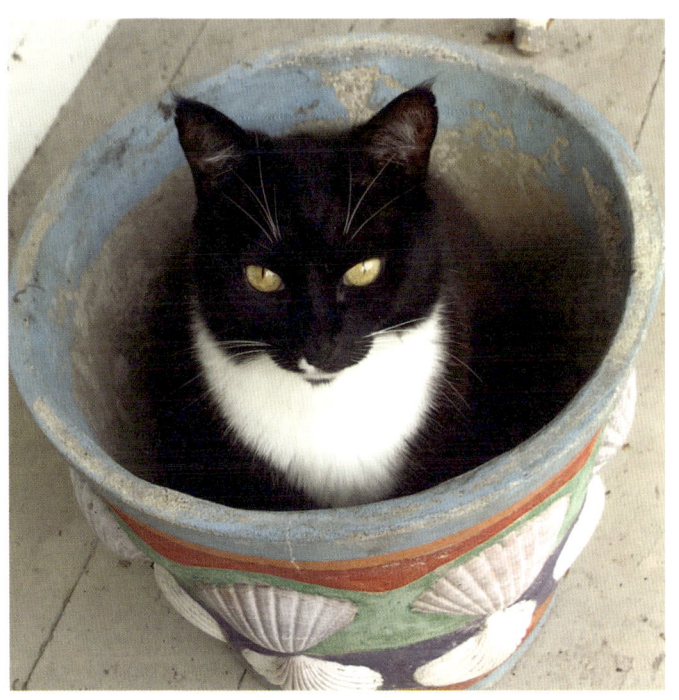

against agony and despair, she was my familiar, and a friend in my moments of panic. Stroking her fur calmed me, centred me, caused my heart rate to lessen its mad gallop. She listened to my fervent prayers and, by remaining mute, she seemed to answer them. To cat loathers I'm aware this will be seen as syrup and misapprehension. Yet to me Parky was a vital part of my life, a survival strategy. And now she is gone.

How unfathomable is the relationship between animal and human? Did I imagine her affection? Did I anthropomorphise her into cuteness? Why did she come to sleep by my legs but carefully leave a space so she did not harass by touch? Didn't she look directly into my eyes and close her eyes in sequence? She came only to me; she heard my internal voice. We bonded, imperfect needy human and tamed wild cat. We formed a symmetry invisible to others but palpable to ourselves.

I struggle with the vacuum her death delivers. I register only the acuteness of pain, the abruptness of something snatched from me too soon.

And there is my naked hurt. I cry out: Why now, you cruel fucking god, when I need her most?

Listen to the absurdity of a human mourning a cat.

This is a photo of Parky as odalisque, possessing that unique ability of a cat to pose to maximum effect.

January 16, 3.27 a.m.

I set off on my pilgrimage to the oncology clinic in the spirit of my first day at school, with associated nerves and too much baggage (in every sense of the word).

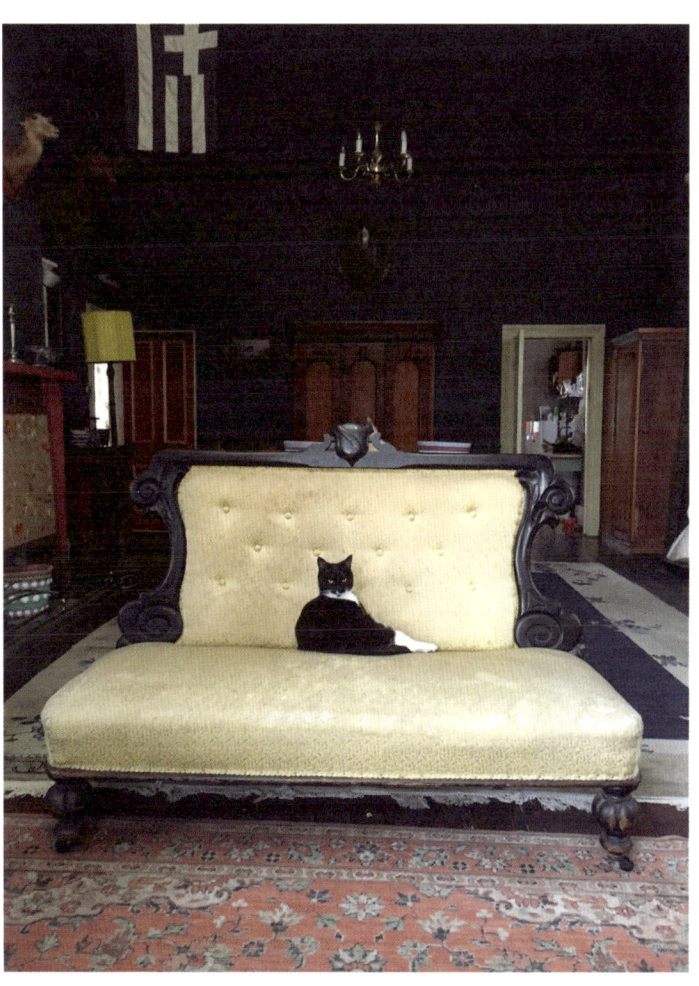

The clinic is a kind of discreet airport lounge for the select (and sick), and several others were being chemicalised behind screen-like barriers. I was led to my own comfy lounge seat with, it was revealed later, semi cocktail-cabinet openings for tea and snacks, plus a screen. I put my books and mags at my feet, while loyal D sat opposite me, and so began the experiment.

I was in a high state of nervous anticipation and it took a long two hours 35 minutes to break me down into lethargic acceptance that I was attached to a machine feeding some sort of chemical substance (Docetaxel – a friend described it as Roundup) into my veins.

At one point, before it all began, there was a mind-blowingly toxic smell, but it quickly went away. My veins were flushed, I was given a steroid, then I too was chemicalised. (The injection was on my right hand just above my wrist, which made it exceedingly difficult to type.)

I sat there in a miasma of boredom, stuck, as it felt, on some sort of eternal long-distance flight. I flicked through the *London Review of Books* and was pleased to note the real title for Oscar Wilde's *De Profundis* was actually 'A Letter from Prison and In Chains'. I then turned to *Metro* for light relief and info on a city I seem to occupy only tangentially, in that it is the city of my birth, a city I love, but which seems to bear little resemblance to the smart restaurants and bars *Metro* describes – though I recognise the highly competitive banter as an Auckland note. Then suddenly Cecil Beaton called me.

I opened it at random (*The Unexpurgated Beaton – Cecil Beaton's Diaries As He Wrote Them*). He was complaining about some sort of hormonal treatment he was having (following the removal of his prostate), how it interfered with

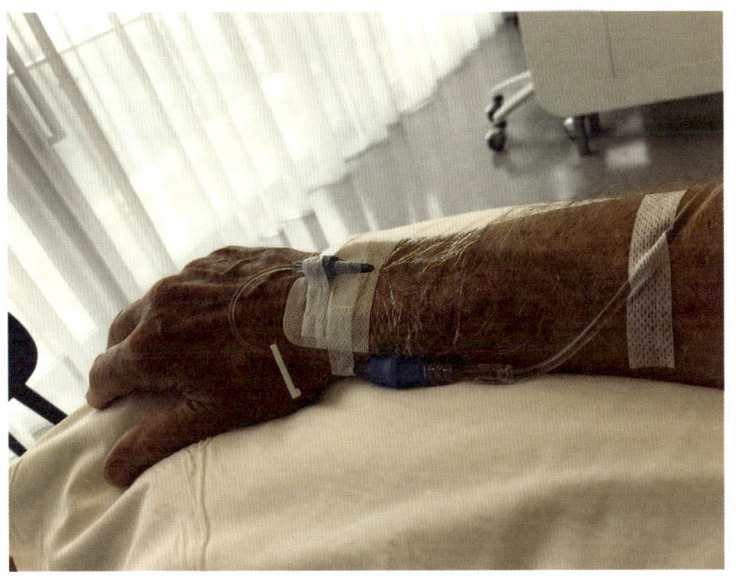

his sex drive (he was slightly older than me) and how his cock had shrivelled to the point he could no longer hold it to piss.

This was more interesting. He diarised the Duke of Windsor's funeral, which I cross-referenced with the *Crown* episodes I'd just seen the night before in which the Duke tries to mock the coronation for his smart cocktail friends but ends up being deeply moved. His funeral was the same – Beaton never liked the Duke but ended up moved by the peerless ancient ceremonial, delivered with a dusting of gossip: the French aristocrats who were scandalised 'a grocer' got better seats than them, the Duchess of Windsor ruthlessly smart but lost in space. I was delighted to see he used 'stink' as we do in conversation – as in 'That was a stink party.' I always thought this was Māori usage.

But oh how the hours leered at me on the long-distance flight. It was a slow patch. There's only one way to cope and that's to go with it. You fade out. You can't believe the sachet of liquid chemical isn't empty. You accept you're in some sort of science-fiction movie, in a set made by TVNZ's *Gloss* department. At times various beepers go off. You sit there attached to a machine, incapable of moving.

Eventually it ends.

The human pin cushion is allowed to go home. In a mirror you catch sight of yourself and you're surprised to see you're dramatically pale, almost green – the colour of dirty note paper. You don't feel any different. Just depleted. Worn thin. You've taken the nausea medication and there's more to come. There's the needle you will stick in your belly 24 hours away, tomorrow, 'to bolster immunity'.

That's it. Your first chemo session. You're free to go home, baby.

Outside I'm stunned to find a swarthy hot day alive with wind. The city is still half empty because of the holidays, and the schools you pass have an almost yearning loneliness to them, as if they can't wait to come alive again with the shouts and cries of one thousand children.

You get home and Ajax the cat slinks out of the shade. His fur feels hot. He lies down to be stroked. I say, 'I'm going to lie down. Come inside and lie down beside me. Keep me company.'

I find the bed and I lie down on it like it's a ship that's going to take me home. I close my eyes and relax.

January 17, 6 p.m.

Today I had to give myself an injection in the stomach. I know diabetics do this daily without so much as a blush. But somehow I've retained a child-like horror of needles (which makes it somewhat ironical I've ended up being a human pin cushion, as I wrote yesterday. But that's with other people handling the needle.) There was no alternative. D said he could not do it. This left me. I always imagine things are worse than they turn out to be (like chemo itself actually). In fact I gave a yell of pain before the needle slid in. It was a tiny diabetic needle and it was into belly fat. There was almost no sensation at all. I pushed the needle flange down. It was over. I felt curiously elated. I had done something I had never done before in my entire life. I felt like laughing with glee.

January 19, 3.42 a.m.

It was as if I walked into a wall. The morning had gone exceptionally well and I drew up a list of things I wanted to do – a walk by the sea, a book I wanted to order at Wardini's book store, some tickets for Prima Volta. In fact I was feeling so energised I decided to print some photos of Parky. I had also made a note to go and collect Parky's ashes.

Physically I seemed to be defying the chemo slump (though it was only two days in, and usually it occurs between days seven and ten). Then suddenly about midday I felt my energy drain out of me. It was astonishingly fast, as if someone had pulled a plug on an air mattress then forced all the air out.

I decided to do a few things regardless. I found myself not walking but wading through air. At the supermarket I had so little energy I didn't let the woman who had only two items to purchase go ahead of me – I just stood there obstinately with my shopping trolley. Then the very sobering business of picking up Parky's ashes at the vet. There was a small wooden box. Her name was engraved on the front. I looked at it and thought, From this (a live cat full of contradictions and mystery) to this (a tiny box of inert matter). Is that what it amounts to? A little box full of blood and bone? Yet I clung even to the ashes. If that was all that was left of her, I would accept them as the closest I would ever be – could ever be. Such morbidity. Such sentimentality. Yet it isn't. It is a sober and sobering gaze – at the remains of a cat.

The good news is my new book *Dear Oliver* is hurtling out into the bookshops in March. It was to come out in May, which seemed to me forever away, kind of like a trek to Moscow through the snow. So the news that it is coming out earlier really pleases me.

What is the book about? Its subtitle covers it very well: 'Uncovering a Pākehā history'. It's an exploration of Pākehā-tanga through the colourful stories of one family (my mother's family) – how they triumphed, how they failed, the stories they told. I'm the guide, so it's all in my voice. And it's framed with the source of all my family stories – my redoubtable mother, Bess.

The book is also framed by my looking after her in her final years, so the territory oddly enough is not too different from what I'm writing now – introspective, reflective, discursive, musing on life and death.

I've always thought Pākehā are the least examined of people in contemporary Aotearoa, the most casually dismissed and overlooked. Not exotic enough, lacking a triumphalist narrative (overcoming hardship to reach acceptance): it's an under-explored territory. And I've chosen the highly personal lens of my own family to tell the story.

It frightens the hell out of me now we're getting close to publication. When I got the first copy of the book my reaction, on seeing so many photos of my family, was to slam it shut in an impulse of shame. 'How can you betray your family by telling all its secrets?' This is a paraphrase of my mother's voice, which I can hear in my head as I type. It's hard to answer except to say, I don't have much time left, Mum. I'm on the final lap. It's now-or-never territory and a lot of these stories I've lived with, in my head, all my life. Besides, I'm an historian. I am trained to wield the scalpel of truth. I am also your child, so I have an inherent loyalty to fables I was nourished on. End result – the kind of creative conflict which hopefully produces a good book.

The bad news is . . . March is probably when my hair will fall out. I will have had my second chemo by then. OK, I am vain. I have an ordinary human's interest in presenting a reasonable version of myself. Especially when 'in the public eye'. Instead I will be the most reduced, the most humiliated I will ever be (so far, a horrid little voice chirps). That is, I will be bald. I will be to some extent reduced, showing evidence of what I'm going through. Live with it, some other voice in my head says. Get used to it, sister.

January 22, 2.27 a.m.

Every picture tells a story. This is the 1973 Graduate Parade up Queen Street. Helen Clark and I were chosen to lead the MA graduates. I particularly like this photo because Mojos is in the background. I'm wearing a second-hand brown herringbone tweed suit with a green tartan tie and, out of shot, my brown two-tone (caramel and brown) platforms (hence why I tower over Helen).

Mojos was where we went to get a taste of real life; it was where 'drag queens', as we called them then, hung out and performed. Fiona Clarke took photos there. So it's a kind of

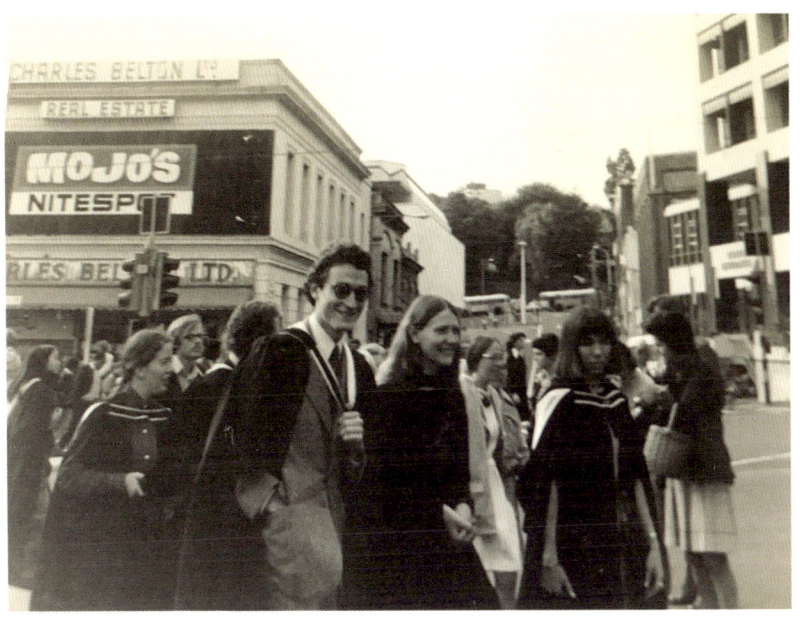

daylight shot which alludes to a seamier night-time reality in which I partly lived. I have Tuinal churning through my system from the night before. It's a barbiturate. It was the '70s after all. I was also about to enter a time I would always look back to with fondness. And this was a sort of golden period in which I knew I was going away to an English university but I had to wait for the September term to start. This gave me, effectively, part of a year in which to play and party – and say goodbye.

I was 23 and I felt I was about to go away forever. I certainly sensed my life was about to change (which it was). So I had a strange irradiance around me: the radiance of someone going away, someone who was about to disappear, but someone who had been 'chosen' too. There was also the implied decadence of a person not doing anything . . . except, in a series of lengthy parties and night-time affairs, saying an extended goodbye. It was during this period that I 'discovered' Auckland. In saying goodbye I consciously looked at Auckland and its inner city as if I were recording it in my mind in advance. I harvested impressions of Auckland as if I really was going away forever. This is when an emotional map was laid – one that led me many years later to attempt to save the Civic, for example. It was like, just when I was leaving New Zealand, I fell in love with it.

But it also felt as if I was living in a lost world. There was a sense of it cresting towards a beautiful impossibility. The fragile constructions on which we built our lives would in time be revealed almost viciously. We all lived, on the surface, in a glow of drugged euphoria, from party to party. Beneath this was another colder, much harsher world. So in that sense the world I was in was already 'lost': it was just we did not appreciate it then. We lived in the last rays of a '70s sunset.

So here I am walking up Auckland's main street with Helen Clark, in my platforms, happily chatting away, on my way off into a future like everybody's future – one I knew nothing about.

Later:
Peg the cat drops by to give me some animal kindness on a day I feel absolutely lousy.

January 23, 4.01 a.m.

It's so depressing when you seem to go backwards. Last night I suddenly got a terrible pain in my lower right back. Instantly all my gains vanished. I was back to square one. I returned to the absolutism of pain. Pain is a complete tyranny that insists it not only owns your body but actually is your body. You can't answer back.

I was back to Ronnie's 'Where's the pain between numbers one to ten?' Despite or because of the absence of pain which led me to abandon my walking stick/crutches for the most part, the searing pain down my right lower back indicated to me I had better: 1) go back to using crutches as a precaution and 2) go back on Sevredol. Sevredol is quick, effective and often lets me obscure the pith of pain by falling asleep. It usually lasts three hours approx. Yet . . . and this is a big yet, it's heavily chemical, leaves me feeling dull and drugged, and like all those pharmaceuticals, slightly depressed. You're down.

On the other hand there are natural alternatives. I've had two friends who have helped me get marijuana to make into biscuits or, alternatively, into a form of butter. Both forms are illegal. It's one of those idiotic things that a country in which marijuana is widely used regards the medical uses of marijuana – surely the most benign form there can be – with an almost medieval suspicion. From my understanding, medical marijuana is available here on prescription but only for the most painful terminal (i.e. deathbed) situations, and then it comes from Canada and is costly. What a farce. Why are we pretending marijuana is some foreign drug about which we all know nothing? Marijuana has been a foundation drug in NZ since at least the 1970s. I'm not sure of figures but people who smoke marijuana or have smoked marijuana must be in the majority. The funny thing is, I'm not really interested in the recreational use of marijuana. At all. (I used to be, though that's another story.) But I am really interested in its use as a solvent against pain, as a relaxant. It's particularly useful against nausea during chemo.

The other day I had a good old-fashioned marijuana chocolate biscuit and I can tell you it offered me an afternoon of complete relaxation as I listened to music. There was a gaudy Saint-Saëns symphony on the radio but I listened as if I had not heard music before. Nothing else existed. Not pain. Not the human body. Not even my niggling querying chattering consciousness. What's the harm in that? I just want marijuana used for medical purposes to be freely available to those in pain. It's so obvious it's hard to see why it needs stating.

January 24, 5.21 a.m.

How do you tell people? How do you tell people you have cancer? I was struck with this problem this morning in Georgia, a coffee place I go to each morning I'm in Napier. I had a crutch, which is always a red flag. 'So what's wrong?' an acquaintance asked, mid-conversation. I quickly computed the circumstances. It was a casual inquiry, equivalent to 'How are you?' (Don't answer, I couldn't care less.) So I stammered out, 'I've got a back problem', thinking that isn't entirely inaccurate. This seemed to answer the immediate inquiry, though it left the Protestant truth-teller in me full of uneasiness. My friend vanished none the wiser.

But I've had the experience before, in similar circumstances, of answering, 'I've got cancer', only to find the recipient of such news incapable of giving a response. Her reply was virtually 'That's nice,' though what she meant was 'That's devastating, I can't take it in, let's talk further at some other stage.' One acquaintance said, 'Bummer', which I thought was entirely inadequate to the circumstances. I was offended.

It's really hard to walk the line between sententious, precious and straightforward. You have to feel for what's right in the circumstances. For example, at Georgia's today I found myself spontaneously saying, 'I'm having chemo and my taste buds have all changed' when explaining why I had changed from a longstanding order of a latte to a cappuccino. (The staff had been fobbed off with the bad-back excuse at the beginning.) This was a perfectly smooth introduction to the difficulties of the truth. The young woman who served instantly looked sympathetic. She didn't say anything immediately but later asked quietly, 'Are you having to go to Palmerston North?'

(for chemo). I felt so relieved. I had managed to deliver a difficult truth – or really an awkward truth – but in such a way it didn't rip open the surface of the day. Life went on but with a changed computation about why I was using a crutch – why I might look bad on certain days.

It's all how it plays on the day, on the circumstances, which you have to judge quite quickly. You have to fight back, on bad days, the impulse to say, 'It's none of your fucking business.'

January 25, 3.36 a.m.

Some things my mother taught me:

One could almost say my mother's dying taught me how to live. I was close by her in her final years and I observed her ability to survive in difficult and painful circumstances. She drew on inner resources that kept her, on the whole, remarkably civil and even at times cheerful. She was quick to make a joke out of a situation, even if it was at her own expense. She was uniformly pleasant to the people trying to help her. She understood the difficulties of their jobs, that they weren't paid much and struggled alike to maintain their dignity in an unequal situation. There were times of course when her patience ran out or her pain was so bad that she could barely speak. But there was a carefulness, a humanity which helped mediate what could otherwise have been a grim situation.

I was not conscious of learning or even looking. The thought that I myself would be in a similar situation so very soon never crossed my mind. I remember now exactly where I was in the street in Napier after Bess had died and her estate was sorted and I thought to myself, Now the future is yours. You have only freedom ahead. You have fulfilled the role of a dutiful son.

How the gods must have laughed. Within five months I was aware something was really wrong, and within six I was told I had advanced metastatic cancer for which there was no cure. How fortunate was I that I could turn – without thinking, without any conscious effort – to the manners I had observed unknowingly. I had been inducted into a school of behaviour which amounted to: a lesson in how to conduct your own death.

I hasten to add there is much more to come that stands outside this narrow orbit: what happens to me, how it goes; whether I defy statistics; unlearn what I was given. Yet to me the gradual possession of a kind of wisdom was the best part of an inheritance from a mother I loved – a woman the medical profession defined as 'a dementia patient' (page 150). How could wisdom and dementia sit side by side? Call that one of the great mysteries but I have seen it.

January 29, 5.13 a.m.

I have a problem. It's to do with taking my pills. My subconscious absolutely refuses to accept I have to take pills four times a day. I'll do anything rather than take them. Most of all, 'forget'. But how can you forget something on which your health is partly based? It's not that onerous, swallowing a number of pills (nine for breakfast, for example, these days).

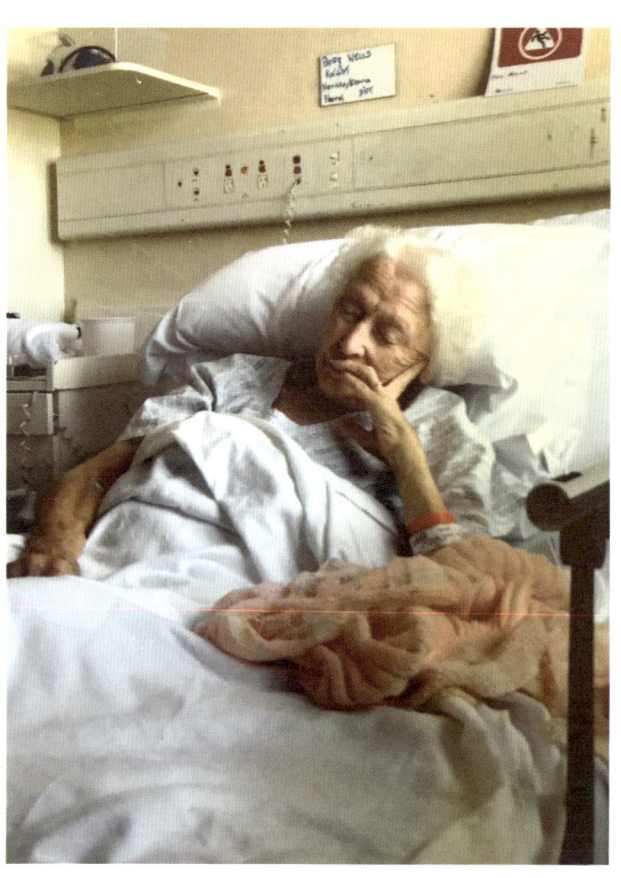

But every day I go through the same fundamental struggle. Every meal is blighted by their presence, their horrible acrid taste. Yet really it's not so bad. If you get a chemical whiff as they go down you can eat a nice ripe plum or a kiwifruit afterwards. Besides, I've mastered the art of quaffing multiple pills: to wit, chuck them all in your mouth dry, take one large glass full of water, take a huge gulp so your mouth is flooded, and somehow the pills float down your gullet. Two swallows at most.

But that's not even it. It's much more basic. It's like: I don't want to take that medicine. I'm sick of taking that medicine. When will it end? Really, I want to deny the fact that I'm sick. In some fundamental way I refute it.

So my subconscious mind is always looking to trick me. Subtly it whispers, Let's do something really clever – let's forget to take your pills this breakfast. Why not just enjoy the flavour of porridge and yoghurt and fruit plus a spanking hot cup of tea. Yes, just relax. It won't take long. And so . . . I run away on a Billy Bunter holiday. My conscious mind meanwhile dons a Mary Poppins pinny and says in crisp tones, Sit up straight, Peter. Is that a curve in your backbone? Let's inspect your fingernails. Now what's this I hear about you not taking your pills?

I know I have to take them. I know my continued health is completely dependent on them. I guess it's just human to want to kick over the traces, to pretend you are actually free of the plaint that dogs you at every step. And in that lies the nutshell. I'm never going to be free. Not really. It's just part of my current adult life that I have to . . . accept a bitter pill, or pills.

Do I believe I am going to die in the next few years? Some part of me has to be prepared for this. Metastatic prostate cancer that has entered the bones is notorious for its ruthless speed. (I googled it and it said that once it enters the bones most men have less than two years to live. Is Google to be trusted, however?)

But do I think I will somehow be excepted? Yes, in some deep prehistoric part of my brain I feel I will not die. This is the spoilt me, the prima donna me, the one who calls out: SURELY NOT ME! ANYONE BUT ME! I feel deeply offended by the idea.

Well, why then this literary pose that you are close to dying or at least intimate with the idea? Am I being counterfeit, maximising public sympathy, milking it while secretly having tickets on the fact I might be alive in twenty years' time, boring everyone senseless? It's so hard to work out, and in that lies the precise problem. No one will tell me 'how long I've got'. At times I feel astonishingly strong and vital. The blood of my peasant ancestors pours through my veins. I will live forever, I feel, when I'm like this. But it only needs the smallest upset and my vulnerability is pathetically revealed. The curtain slides up almost with malevolence. I gaze on the theatre of death, the characters welcoming me in. 'Not yet,' I cry out. 'Give me some more time. I need . . . I need to do . . . (anything almost so long as I can stay alive).'

So what am I? A counterfeit personality milking the public's sympathy? An emotional carpetbagger, a liar? Or someone confused about exactly where he stands? Maybe I'll be doing handstands in ten years' time. I just don't know.

(When the Manaaki Programme pamphlet arrived from Mercy Hospice I felt a sense of complete disbelief, almost outrage, when I saw a sub-bracket termed 'Planning Ahead'. It read, 'Funeral Planning'. I just looked at it and gasped. Surely this doesn't mean me? Am I meant to be planning my funeral already?)

I do, however, try and live looking in two directions – forwards and . . . not backwards (though I enjoy looking into the past, which reveals itself as unexpectedly rich: I seem to understand it better, I feel through the layers to a personal truth that eluded me before). But I also look into a dark unknown, trying to make myself a little more familiar with its shape. Bess, my mother, helped me there, though I have no illusion that dying isn't messy, chaotic, dirty. After all, it is decomposition, reduction. It is removal, ultimately. Does it help to live so openly on the page? Yes, it does. It helps me to speak. I don't want to be frightened by a noisy silence. I'd rather gabble. I'd rather sing. I'd rather do almost anything than face that long dark frozen silence ahead.

January 29, 6.12 a.m.

There is the old saying, You can't go home again (Thomas Wolfe). But you can travel back, not as a tourist exactly, but as an older mortal – and one aware of his mortality. I'm talking about going back to Point Chev where I grew up. Some friends live right on the beach in an elegant residential development. When I was a child in the 1950s it was a vast dark stinky changing shed – we were forbidden to enter as bad things happened there, as well as 'diseases'. But it was also the site of all childhood desires: the ice-cream shop. There was no greater pleasure than lying on your back in a warm salty sea and licking a buttery ice cream which was running down your fingers even as you licked. The salt of the sea melded with the sugariness of the ice cream, a perfect sweet-sour mix.

As children who lived right by the sea we were arbiters of the tides and, most of all, those strange forlorn times when the Point was no longer a holiday destination but went back to being a forgotten unfashionable back suburb of Auckland.

How you relate to where you grew up changes with age. As I became adolescent I hated it with the scalded feelings of someone who had been brutalised. It was, as they say, the site of an original trauma. I forgot the tide, the special quality of living on a distant isthmus, which was Pt Chevalier's peculiar quality – suburban but also almost lunar, certainly forgotten. I avoided it all and imaginatively grew up somewhere else. (Anywhere else, hence books and films and stories and make-believe.)

It took me many years to come to terms with living in Pt Chev, or rather with what happened when I lived in Pt Chev, and this occurred when I was as far away from it as I could physically get. It was in the dismal chill of pre-Thatcherite Britain that the warmth and strange lullabies of a Pt Chev childhood came back to haunt me. Soon enough I could not think of anything else. My subconscious had triumphed. Eventually this would lead me home to NZ, to reappraise my whole emotional relationship to 'home'.

Part of this reappraisal was writing my first novel *Boy Overboard*, which is both a rapt description of a world eerily like Pt Chevalier but also an attempt to untie some psychological knot that had held me trussed all my adult life (OK, 'fucked

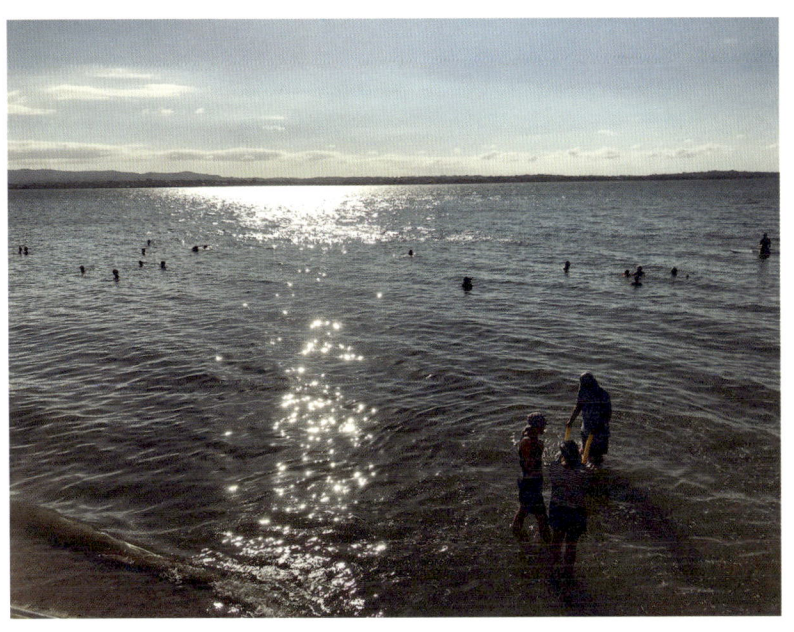

me up' in contemporary parlance). Bad things had happened to me in my Pt Chev youth – as bad things happen to us all as we stumble through life, especially as unguarded kids. The psychological tightness of the 1950s is something we tend to forget – all those men fucked up by killing in war having to come home and settle down, all those women who had to forget the sweet taste of freedom they'd experienced when 'the men went away'. It was the time of the Cold War, of spies, suspicion and nuclear Armageddon. So my experience of Pt Chev took in not only the familiarity of Coyle Park and the running club and church at the Ascension, and every Saturday going up the road to the flicks, but also this other more complex layering both psychological and, one might say, global.

Yet if there was one thing that could recall me to the sweeter aspects of my childhood it was the water – the tide. It has something slightly sacred about it, as it recalls my now vanished brother and mother and family, my best friend Jackie and another whole tribe of local connections. It's also more practically the tide – a place to swim – and if it so happens that every tree, every stone eerily recalls the past, so be it. It's deeply detailed but, more beautifully, it is just itself – it's what it is.

And this is what I'm most looking forward to experiencing when I go out to visit these kind friends: I'm going home to a place which is no longer home but which will always be the place I came from, the place I was formed, the place I ran away from – and the place to which I returned.

January 30, 3.19 p.m.

It suddenly occurred to me I was having too much of a good time. Here I was in the car, racing in to have a wig consultation, radio blasting songs from my high-period youth – 'Gimme Shelter' (turned up extra-loud as I was in the car alone), then that old pious anthem 'Something in the Air' (the Revolution's near).

I felt positively hilarious with a frail kind of happiness. What was wrong with me? I had cancer, didn't I? What did I think I was doing? Hair loss from cancer is a serious issue. It's not a game, something to trifle with. But I was intent on seeing what a wig could 'do for me' in case of hair fallout from my second chemo.

The hair place was on a small side street off Upper Queen Street and I had a 9.30 a.m. appointment with Kylie. Kylie turned out to be a super-energetic wig consultant. She explained to me there are only two wigs for men – the usual lack of choice based on gender. But she explained to me how she could trim and cut them back so they weren't so fulsome.

I was interested in being experimental. A Warhol-style wig at one point appealed. But really they only had two bog-standard male wigs, only one of which was in the silver-white range.

Time to try it on.

Kylie professionally got it on my scalp and it felt OK. But when I looked in the mirror I burst out laughing. She said that was OK. Her last client laughed and laughed and laughed. Well, it's either that or crying.

So here it is, the evidence of my wig-out. I think I look like a Bay of Plenty radio personality up on a morals charge. I don't quite look like me.

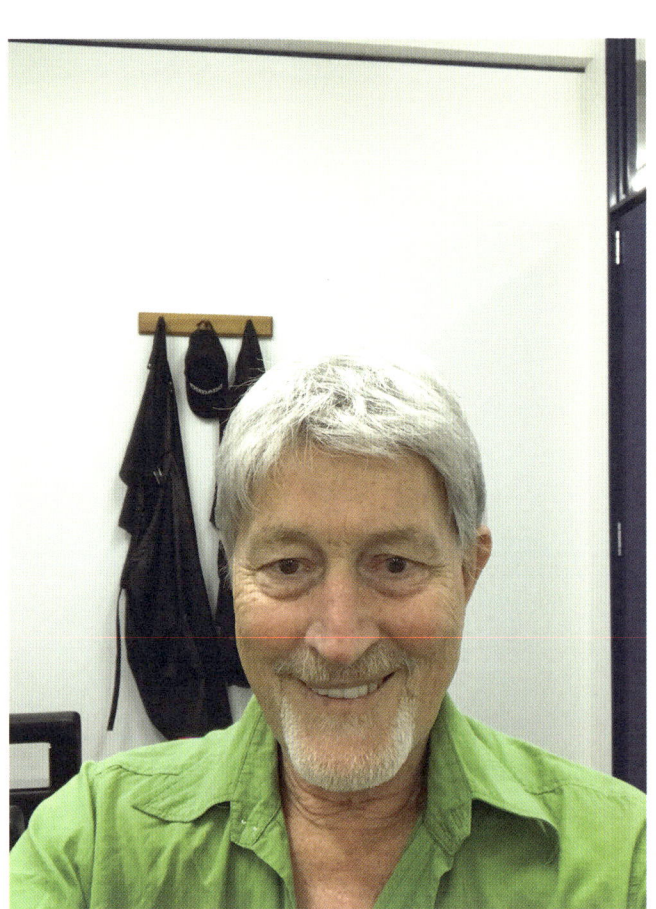

Kylie has assured me she's a mastermind with the scissors and it is, after all, a kind of therapeutic service aimed at helping people suffering from hair fall-out from chemotherapy. It's actually a very serious business. But I'm pleased, in the photo, I'm so cheerful.

31 January 2018, 7.10 a.m.

Wading into the tepid salty sea at Pt Chev I realised I now had the body of an older man, of the kind that I used to glance at when I was a child playing in the shallows. These bodies seemed somehow fantastic, grotesque, almost impossible to compute with your own. They were all accretion, collapse. There was no beauty there, or athleticism. The most that you could hope for was a gravity, almost a dignity, of persistence through time. In my childhood these older men and women often wore wool bathing suits. They were shockingly bad. They sagged even when dry. Once wet, they went in almost science-fiction deformations. But my point here is that I had at long last joined a parade of ancients from whom physical beauty was hidden.

Not that the beach at the Point was a parade of beauty. There were all sorts of body types, of ethnicities, a lot of cheerily overweight people. At times it felt like the Middle East, with a kind of up-close eroticism accompanied by music playing loudly and, I noted, vodka and beer. Point Chev was never a classy beach. It had once been the beach for landlocked Ponsonby and Grey Lynn, when people either bussed out or came in huge old 1940s cars, carrying blankets and thermoses.

But what concerns me here is my graduation into that invisibility as an older man. Sure, I saw my younger self there, playing amid the waves. There were so many earlier versions of myself there. Wasn't I lucky anyway to make old bones – even bones as old as these? Hadn't lots of friends dropped off along the way, vanishing in that abrupt way that left you staggered that they were no longer there? You had to be grateful for what you had, as I was, wading out over the flat long shelf of sand which is a peculiarity of all tidal beaches. I noted one or two male beauties, a few curvaceous women showing themselves off in a way that would once have been deemed 'shameless'. Yet can beauty know shame?

I don't think so. It's one of the things I'm having to get used to – losing vanity, coming to terms with mortality. This is part of the ageing process anyway, but I had hoped to be of that older generation that did not so much defy age, as try to deploy whatever arts one had, to 'make it fun', stylish. Now I realised there was a bottom line: I was lucky to be alive. I was very lucky to be alive. I could luxuriate in something as simple as going for a swim. (As for going for a swim in a place redolent with childhood associations – that's caviar.) This comes under the heading of a motherhood saying: 'Be grateful for what you've got.'

It's true for that ageing old dripping candle of a body wading out to sea too. I can still walk, I can still swim. It's that pervasive feeling I've had ever since I got told that I had this blasted cancer. I'm lucky on so many levels – not on the level of cancer, of course, not at all. But somehow at times I seem to be so vividly alive – it's not chemicals, I think. It's not drugs (or if it is, get me more). It's just I see life now as a holiday. I just can't explain it any other way. All the old rules are gone.

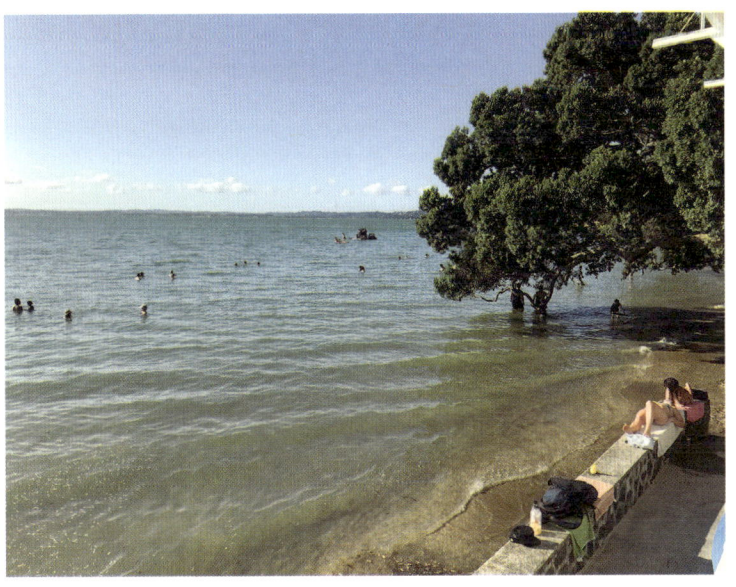

The calendar has been ripped to shreds. Time has a different meaning. And today I'm not in pain, today I'm perfectly OK. So let me explain it no further. I'm happy.

February 3, 4.26 a.m.

This is a self-portrait/selfie I took on 21 November 2017 in my office in Greenlane. The results were finally in. I was out of hospital and I had been given the medical information, most of which was so esoteric I struggled to understand it. '*Newly diagnosed met prostate ca, Gleason 9, PSA 100*'. Then there was other information which terrified me. '*There is widespread metastatic disease throughout the spinal column. There is involvement in all vertebrae with abnormal T1 and T2 signals.*'

I knew I had a disease for which there was no cure, that the disease was advanced – very advanced – and that I was in some sense in a critical situation. This is really a photograph of me facing my mortality. My stare is unflinching, even unsparing (or is the effect of morphine giving me a slightly mad stare?). Behind me recedes my life – the mirror on my office wall, then, through the door, the calm of a domestic setting, a sitting room with a lamp and a cabinet. My hair still has some colour, my eyebrows have the black hair which was the only place on my body I ever had black hair. (They are now white.) I do not appear distressed. Rather I'm thoughtful, trying to work out the meaning of the situation in which I so suddenly find myself. I do not look sick. I have looked much worse. But here I present a face to the world which is calm,

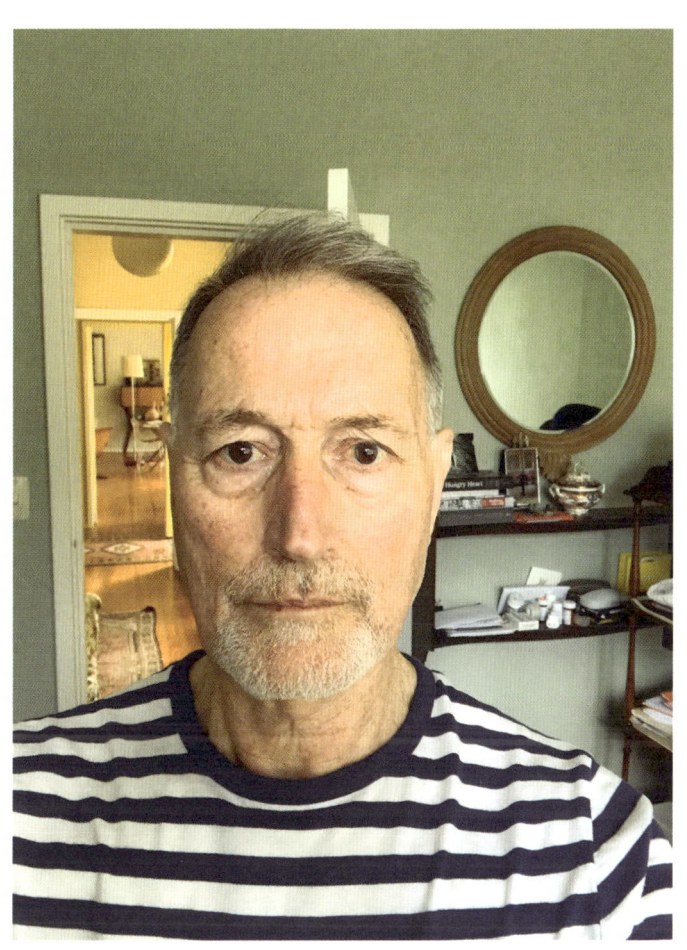

implacable, inquiring – and, inevitably, but screened from the lens, deeply shocked.

I'm pleased I took this photo. It's like my passport photo. As to what foreign country I am travelling to, I'm uncertain. You could call it – my future.

February 4, 7.59 p.m.

It seemed forever ago that I had driven to Ascot Hospital in the early morning to meet the urologist who had kindly agreed to see me before he started meeting clients. Everything seemed in a state of emergency, which I barely failed to appreciate. A few days later he delivered the news that I had incurable cancer and that I needed immediate and urgent treatment.

As I drove past the building today I felt distant from it all, yet almost nostalgic, which is a most peculiar emotion for something so stark. By this I mean, I felt I was treated well and decently and everything that flowed from that moment had been done well. What this is about is the small grace of human contact which does so much to make 'a life in medicine' bearable.

Today I was having my bloods and testosterone read before my Monday chemo – my second round. The woman who took my blood was a migrant, efficient, personable, just into early middle age. You are only ever in the room alone for a few minutes but in that time we managed to establish a rapport. First it started with her skilfully asking a question just before the needle dug in. I was diverted, relaxed. Then we went on to chat further when she showed me the vials of blood for me to confirm that they carried my correct name and birthdate. I wasn't wearing my glasses and this led to some badinage about declining sight with age, all of it light and humorous. We parted almost like friends. Of course not real friends. But somehow the humanist impulse made what was otherwise routine into something special.

I have come across this so often on my brief medical odyssey. The urologist who had the difficult job of delivering bad news had the mien of a man who regretted what he was doing, but he also had a gravity which bespoke kindness, empathy. Ronnie the nurse was someone I almost fell in love with because she was so worldy-wise and tough but kind. Again and again I brushed up against people who made the small interactions a chance to express the grace of being human. So this post is about looking back quickly at a moment that changed my life. 'What's gone and what's past help/Should be past grief', Shakespeare advises in *The Winter's Tale*, but that's not always easy to obey – I'm not sure I'm past grief. But what alleviates the situation is the human interactions that help you concentrate on the fact you're still alive.

Later, as I drive away, I even conceive the idea I might survive this cancer. I suffer very little pain these days and my meds seem to do whatever they're meant to do. Is it possible I'll survive longer than had been initially thought?

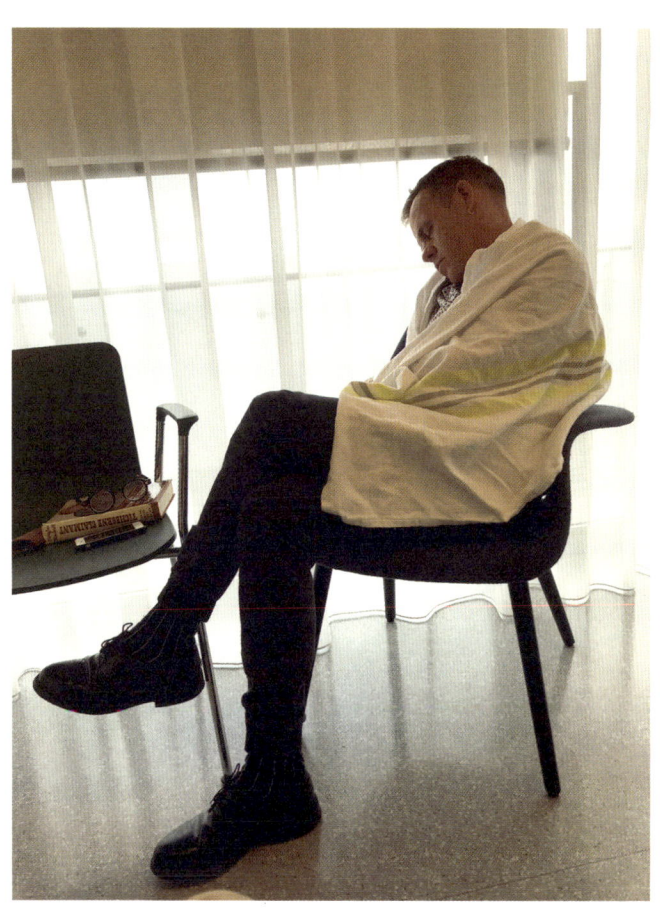

My companion. D sleeps in the chilly room while I have a two-hour chemo session.

February 6, 2.47 a.m.

I'm OK today but a little groggy. I wish I could write less personally but here goes.

The hormone 'therapy' is starting to take effect. My body is changing. My flesh has the strange cheesy colour of old beeswax. My breasts seem bigger (if one can talk of men having breasts). My hair has started to fall out in a quiet almost illicit way, hair by hair. I have to come to terms with decline and change. It's not easy. But there isn't a choice. Or rather there is a choice (stop all treatments) but that is not a real one. Yet the strangest thing is I am not entirely depressed. D has asked me to respect his privacy so I can only talk of this from my POV. But I seem to be coming to a new understanding of things.

It is a key part of gay ideology (or is it general sexual ideology?) that you must be attractive to be loved, to find love. You must be chiselled, thin, etc. Attraction is allegedly based on physical looks above all. This hyper-narcissism so infects our culture that even young All Blacks are struggling to live up to unreal body images.

How very strange to walk through the mirror and find myself steadily losing whatever bodily attractiveness I once had – but to find myself experiencing a deeper, more profound, more peaceful love. This is something I never thought of. I just assumed this was end of the line and one would struggle on as best as one could. It is a strange inverse learning and not without its humbling qualities.

I feel a core of trust and peace that is, of course, different from the rough allure of sexual desire, but in its own way deeply gratifying. I think actually it is an explanation for my unreasonable happiness, against all the odds. This arrived, unbidden, in silence, and is more than I ever expected in my life.

There seems so much to learn in this situation, humility being chief among the mysteries.

12 February

I had to go back to Auckland Hospital today for Radiology to check on my progress. I was unprepared for the emotional weight of being back in those familiar buildings – buildings which time had quickly made into set pieces for my own particular drama. (In my mind I had folded the stage scenery away. It was finished. At least that's the way I felt when I looked at Ascot Hospital so dispassionately the other day.) But there the hospital was, grimy, seemingly eternal. It brought me out into a sweat of dread. Even my breathing changed. (Shallow, quick.) The dread of being back. Of being a captive again in the house of sickness.

We 'followed the green line' in one of those aimless shambles, suddenly passing the space where I was first admitted. I have to admit I felt a quiet burst of horror. (It had that same timelessness, the fixed fluorescent glare. A nurse in a trance slowly walked across the space on the diagonal.

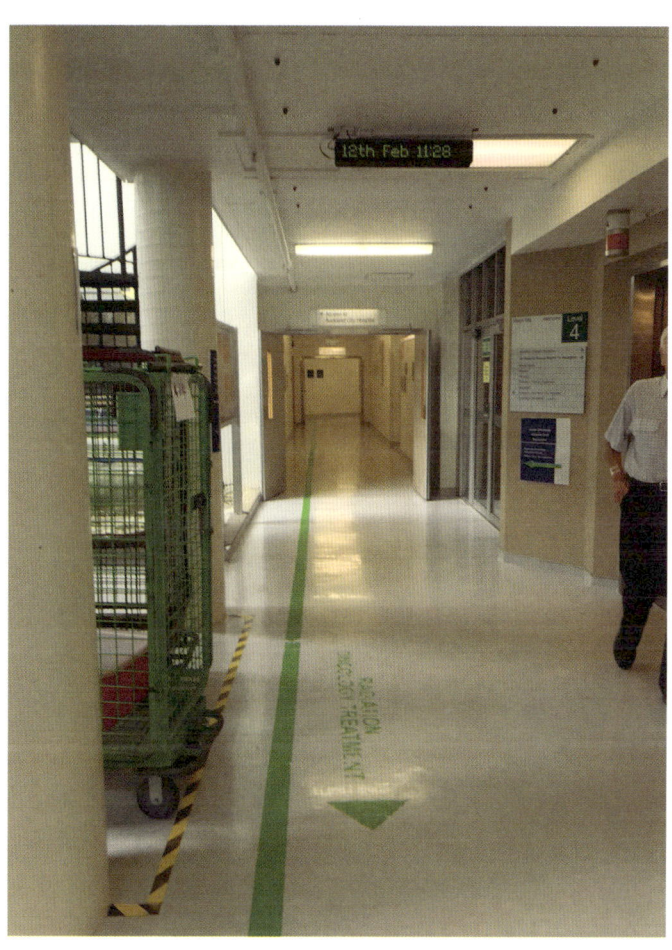

Or was I in a trance?) Then we found the correct waiting room and sat. I went back to that feeling – time no longer belongs to you. You are a petitioner, if not a prisoner. You have no rights (or very few rights). Passivity is the best thing. You sit there. The television runs inanely like a form of contemporary dribble. It's just loud enough to puncture any internal thought. The never-ending nature of it is such that you comprehend the small drama of your health: your improvement, recovery, etc is immaterial, you are to some extent of very little concern in this monolith. But not entirely of no concern. You do – just – matter enough for you to wait, queue, etc. But you're back inside the beast. All its rhythms become your rhythms. Its heartbeat your heartbeat. You're no longer free. Or: the illusion of freedom is taken from you.

Then you are called into the doctor's room. Your doctor is away sick and it's a young doctor there who seems like a bit-player suddenly thrown into the main actor's role. She's not entirely convincing. Besides, it's pretty much a rote check, it turns out. The subtext is: how are you? You OK? No probs with the radiation? Once we establish everything is fine, I'm released. I can go.

Suddenly the swerve towards freedom is so intense I feel an almost rhapsodic happiness overtake me. I suddenly love the doctor, the receptionist, people I see in the corridors. I'm free, I can get away. I practically run down the corridor. I can return to the illusion that I have nothing to do with the hospital, or rather I can wander away without perceiving I am still attached but the string is merely invisible to my eyes . . . but at that moment I don't care.

I get in my car and drive away fast.

Within ten minutes I forget the hospital exists.

February 14, 4.49 a.m.

At what point do you set off on a pilgrimage to a strange and foreign land? I ask this, as two kind friends have sent me information about new prostate cancer treatments, neither of which is available in NZ. One is called Radioisotope Therapy which delivers high doses of targeted radiation to prostate cancer sites while sparing normal tissue. It's also very useful for bone metastases (my problem) where radioactive particles including Strontium-90 are used to blast the site (I'm sure there is a more medical way to term this). It's available in Melbourne and is costly ($10,000 a dose), though it can be done on a single day.

The other is merely a smoke signal on a distant sky. It's a drug called enzalutamide. (Where do these names come from? Is Cruella De Vil in the business of naming drugs on the quiet?) It has not yet been peer reviewed for publication so is a long-distant hope for men like me with cancer in their bones.

I'd heard when a close friend, another Peter, was sick, about these men who are very active in roaming the world in search of the latest treatments and possibilities. There is even a man by the amazing name of Snuffy Myers (resident of Virginia) who is regarded as a sort of karmic leader imbued with almost psychic powers of divination in terms of new treatments. At the time I felt almost a form of pity for these men driven to the ends of the earth in search of a cure. It seemed a statement of the desperation of their case rather than the likelihood of a cure. But now I find myself in a similar state I am not so languid. At the same time, some part of me resists this last-stage attempt at salvation (it's strange how religious metaphors keep cropping up – what does that mean?).

I'm still only midway through my programme of treatment, the three-speared attack through chemotherapy, radiation and hormone treatment – what my urologist, a man of unusually sober temperament, described as 'throwing everything at it'. So far my response has been good. My PSA has gone down from an almost hallucinatory 365 to an acceptable 35. I walk without crutches or stick. I have not so far, touch wood, suffered nausea and other side-effects from chemo. I am greedy for life. But then who isn't?

In terms of further treatments, I have to press pause till the three-headed course ends so we can get a better sense of where I am at. Might I just go on living in some sort of reduced but still possible way? I seemed to enter the game at the most disastrous point, so loaded with disease my frame was almost cracking under the weight of it. Can I continually just get better while never actually getting better? Can I . . . ah, you see, here I am pleading for crumbs, pleading abjectly. It's the same thing that sends these men fanning out to the ends of the earth in search of deliverance/salvation/hope.

I would go on the pilgrimage if I ended up at the Last Hope Cafe. Of course I would try. I'm not sure I would spend the rest of my life trying, however. I have a reality principle embedded pretty deeply within me. I'd rather spend whatever time is left to me enjoying myself rather than sitting in hospitals enduring painful treatments. But we'll see. I have to accept that if I am faced with the fact my treatment has failed (what does that mean precisely? – I knew the limited terms of the contract anyway), if I am told I am going to die soon, and somewhere on a far horizon a smoke signal emerges – would I have the strength of character to ignore it? I think not.

This is a post about the effects of taking Zoladex which reduces the testosterone on which prostate cancer feeds. I write this, knowing it can be construed as revealing. I take the stance that so long as one looks at a thing with the full power of the gaze, humiliation does not enter into the equation.

Chemical castration. Such a profoundly ugly term. I find myself trying to evade the pivot of the cruellest bargain: that one loses one's sexual vitality in order to stay alive.

I have always had a complicated attitude towards sexuality. My natural development was stymied, like so many gay men of my era, by the illegality and stigmatisation of the time. In my own case I had an extra-bonus, you might call it: I was sexually abused as a boy by an 'uncle'. I can barely bring myself to raise the issue. First because it was pretty much endemic to the time, and secondly because I resist the idea that sexual abuse is a rationale for all sorts of later problems in life. It was just something that happened. It was a corrugation of my soul. I became frightened, even terrified of sex. It took many, many years for my feelings to unfurl, or even for me to understand what had happened. For decades it seemed a profound mystery. One moment I was a boy. The next moment I was fucked up.

And when I did unfurl, it was, maybe fortunately, during the years of Gay Liberation. I walked into the future, however, carrying the baggage of the past. (I did not understand this.) It took me many years to relax into something that other people might see as easy and natural and casually accepted. And like so many gay men, once I was free (or freed), I raced ahead barely being able to stop gulping down life's pleasures. I mean here,

173

sex. I needed sex in order to know I was alive. That dead body from childhood which I carried into maturity needed to be not so much buried decently as brought alive, given the grace of some kind of acknowledgement as to what had happened, then to be allowed to fade away in shade and quiet.

As I said, it's complicated.

Only then did I learn to understand myself sexually, which meant, as much, learning to understand other people. People always talk of sex as somehow separated from the rest of life rather than intimately connected with every aspect of it. Who hasn't, after a great experience of sex, felt the world was riven with beauty and meaning and energy? Yes, energy, that most important force.

So what happens when you make a bargain that you will forgo sexual energy in order to simply stay alive? What a knavish, slavish proposition. Yet it is one I have accepted in taking Zoladex, knowing, at the same time, that I have already fully explored all my appetites so at least I feel I do not progress into this strange future full of regrets and half-resolved wishes. But that doesn't mean it is easy or even right.

The castration – such a volatile, shall we say, triggering word for nearly every man on the planet – takes the form of a gradual dialling back of sexual feelings. A sort of blank emerges where before there was jagged electricity. Slowly you lose response – not desire, but you become less interested in the connection between feeling and realisation. It is as if you had retired from the human race. You are in the superannuation of desire category. You still look, you still notice, you still vibrate. But there is no motion, not even the desire for motion, beyond this. I found it quite restful at the start. It seemed startling, novel – a holiday away from the senses. Then a stranger thing happened: things that once evoked desire suddenly became quite neutral, then strangely objectified.

As I texted a close friend, a buddy, 'Such a peculiar feeling, as if an outside skin or shell has fallen off. I can't ever remember feeling this asexual, this neutral – this unpersuaded that cock and arse and all the rest of the mystery isn't the core and rationale for existence – maybe it's good for me. As a breather. Maybe it's all a sort of animal protective like going into hibernation?'

Things started to look very different. Let me give you an example. On my Instagram feed I have a mixture, arranged by what algorithm I do not know, that puts royalty (the Romanovs in their last photographic fluorescence – it seems they had a Box Brownie and took their own selfies), interiors, jewels, men's clothing, cats, Princess Margaret and buff men all together, some coy, others in explicit homosexual attitudes. Once I would have glanced at all this paraphernalia of the senses and been mildly erotically entertained by the porny male images. But now, delivered to the other side of sexual feeling, I gaze at the sexual images more objectively and wonder who finds these over-hirsute, pumped-up, slightly babyish men desirable? I lambast the silliness of the sexual choreography. The things that still evoke desire for me are the frozen moments in the dance of pursuit/penetration and flight/submission – something seems quite real here. But so much else about the sexual dramatics appears fake, as fake as they actually are, of course. But what interests me is the distance I feel from them. I might as well be in another country, watching their *National Geographic* performance of sex.

So I look on it as an outsider, someone who is no longer moved, let alone prompted to turn imagination into action.

It's a strange, rather peaceful world to live in, this one. It's like I'm in an aquarium of the senses, a goldfish floating about, a goldfish with some retention of a memory of the great open sea, of huge cataclysmic waves. So that is my side of the bargain at present. Yes, I have had hot flushes – sweat has run down the back of my neck in sheets. And yes, I have felt muddled, my mind at some low-wattage moment. And yes, I have lost touch with the deepest echoes of desire.

If I am to lose so much, am I to be given life? That is, prolonged life (insofar as a man with metastatic cancer – Gleason score 9 – can be)? Who knows? That's part of the devil's bargain. You hope, you trust, you float away on a becalmed sea, semi-praying. Yet I am not unhappy. Perhaps I am no longer aware of what I do not possess. But I think I know quite accurately what I have lost – what disturbances, what riots, what insanities, what wild improbable ecstasies. I am near enough to the practice of them; their vivid memory still echoes for me – I know the taste on my lips and the sweet-sourness of them. But I am travelling calmly on into unknown seas. At the moment I have to.

Later:

Before I went to bed I read and reread this post, but still I hesitated to post it. Why? Because I felt ridiculous – vulnerable – even pathetic. I had once been a writer well known for his sexually explicit writing which had broken a kind of covert mould that held NZ literature back. Now I was tantamount to a eunuch. Did I really want a lot of people to know what my mother would have said was 'my own private business.' Yet I had reached an impasse. I was terrified of putting the post up but I accepted that if I did not make this information clear I could not go on with this inquiry (seeing the whole posting experience as a form of inquiry into how one conducts one's life or equally one's death). And the fact was, with my diminished life, writing these posts constituted my intellectual life: composing a post, thinking about a post, searching for a subject then refining it into words was what I spent every day doing. It was my life, it had become my life.

I could see no way round it. Yet still my courage failed me and I left it unresolved when I went to bed. (Normally the post would be prepared and ready for sending the following day.) But during the night some maturation occurred in my decision-making: I decided I might as well go ahead. Even more so, unless I went ahead, I faced abandoning, in effect, this inquiry. I could doodle posts on various subjects but they would lack the fundamental seriousness which underlies all these posts. Whether I wanted to or not, it was a gate I had to walk through. So in the early morning while it was still dark – as if the darkness would allow me not to see what I was doing – I got up, quickly went into my room, placed the piece of writing on FB then pressed post.

I'm the luckiest person on earth. I always feel this when I walk into our Napier house. It's really where D and I are truly at home. It's a house we created together: it is our joint being expressed in the form of rooms, decor, furniture, books, art and a cat. We also have a house in Auckland, which I know means we enter that percentage of greedy people who have two houses while many poor people don't even have a house at all. But I thought I'd explain a little about what lies behind me feeling I'm the luckiest mortal alive when the key slides into the lock, the door opens back and I walk into the hall.

Having two houses comes from something I regard as a tragedy. My brother Russell died in 1989, prematurely. He was on the threshold of a brilliant career, wherein his lawyerly skills, combined with his humanity and skill at te reo, would have set him up for the top echelon of a new Labour government. Instead he became HIV at a time of extreme stigma, and he died in disgrace in the eyes of many people. Certainly he himself struggled with the abrupt end of his life (at 41) – an end to his promise. But when he died he left his house in Herne Bay to me and his partner, Chris. So if I was helped financially – as I was – this arose out of something that distorted my life and caused me grief – a wound that never really heals.

(I eventually sold the Herne Bay house so I could pay for D's mortgage on his own house in Greenlane. It also freed me up financially to live my life as I wanted. The income of the average writer is below the unemployment level. Now I could be independent.)

So that is one part of the story. The other part of the story relates to this large Victorian house in Napier. We bought it

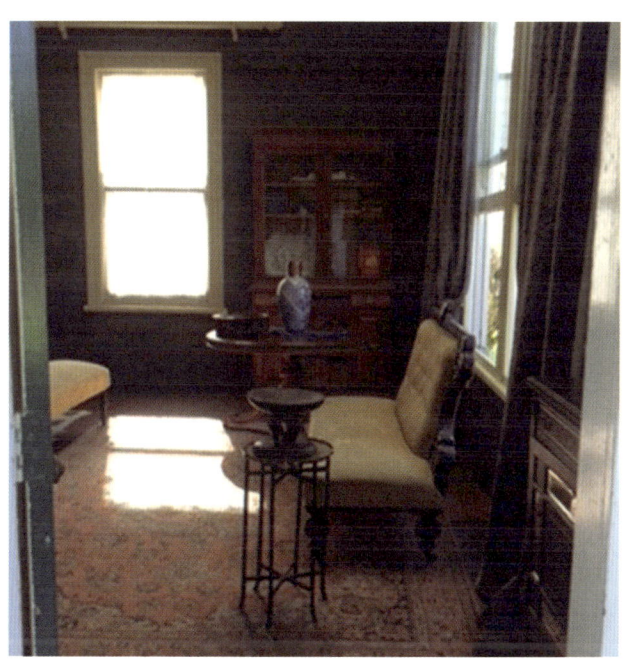

when it was a dump in three flats. I used some of the money from the house in Herne Bay. D had just got a job as director of the Hawke's Bay Museum and Art Gallery. We set to work returning the house to its original glory. It was back-breaking, slow and expensive work but we were fired by a vision. What fun we had going to the local auction house, looking through junk shops. Going to auctions and making heart-thudding decisions to bid. I have to be honest and say this mutual pursuit of an ideal lubricated our relationship, so we sped into the future, fired by mad enthusiasms and ideas. There was always something to find, look at, think about. D is also a contrarian: he was against minimalism and believed in maxi-malism – a drenching of the senses, with scenarios built around atmosphere and a kind of decorative daring.

By the time my mother died I had the furniture and objects which came from my grandmother, my mother and my brother. Instead of being weighed down with a lead sense of obligation, these things were integrated into the maximalist madness. I have a very sentimental attitude to family objects – almost a piety toward them. I like the memory held within a teacup.

Anyway, slowly we built our mad kingdom, our folie à deux. The house here in Napier obliged, flattered to be so buffed up, looked at, thought about. It became our enchanted kingdom.

Then the council decided – and good on them – to develop a new museum and gallery. This was done, but it led to inev-itable cost over-runs and then the inevitable controversy. What happened next was that D became the scapegoat for one of the ugliest things I've ever seen in my life. Basically his career was ruined. The council paid for the ever-duplicitous Wellington consultants to come up to Napier to sing the council's tune: everything was D's fault. D went from being one of the

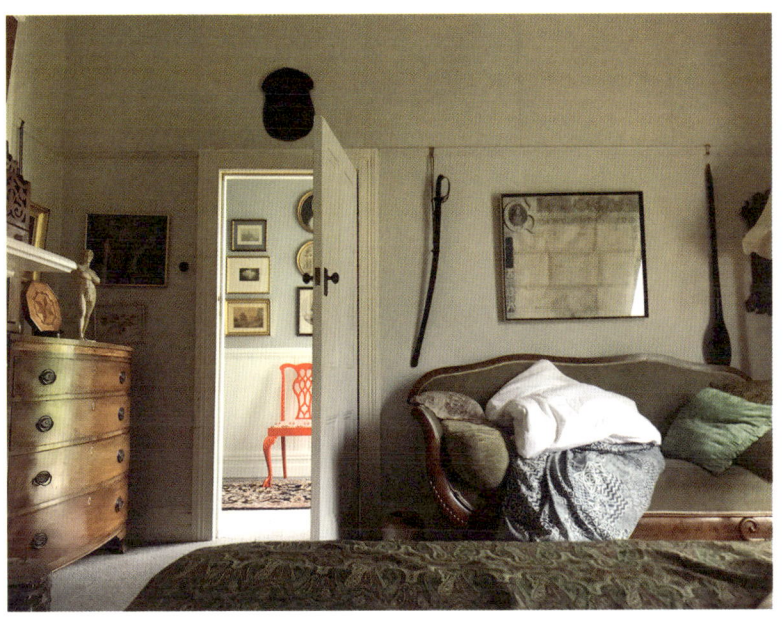

foremost commentators on design and modernism to someone gutted by a callow and bigoted set of provincials intent on one thing only – saving their own arses while making sure D took all the blame. It was ugliness incarnate.

In the end D resigned. Napier became tainted as the site of a disaster. But could we allow those curs to taint our house – our magic kingdom? No. We would not let the bastards destroy that too. We kept on living here, albeit part time, and the magic runes of the house lulled us, soothed us and welcomed us back into a set of values we understood and appreciated. So that is another story which goes towards explaining why I feel I'm the luckiest mortal alive when I walk into the Napier house. There's a whole history there – of survival, persistence, as well as what you might call aesthetic victory, a preference for the hidden mysteries of style over barbarism. And what at first appears as privilege – and I would not deny it is privilege – has to be set beside the fact it is a privilege we've paid for, earned, bitterly at times, against the odds. So privilege too has its price.

As for feeling lucky . . . I know I have cancer and I know I'm in this space – god knows how long it will last – so I might as well enjoy living in this beautiful house which breathes as the soul of two lovers.

February 21, 3.42 a.m.

Letting go. I'm sorting through my papers at the moment for the obvious reason. They've been stacked in the back shed, placed within plastic boxes according to some law of logic which now eludes me. Now each box is dragged onto the back table and I excavate. It's both nauseating and exciting. Nauseating because it's the mess of your past, the turns not taken, the botched plans that never went anywhere, the wryness of wrecked hopes. Exciting because you forget so much – you're forced to forget just to go on living (if we kept full consciousness we'd go mad). But there they are, the tickets to the Biedermeier exhibition you saw in Vienna alongside a Schiele show with a forgotten five-euro note. Or things you'd forgotten like an entire project which never went anywhere even though you had to argue right through to the High Court to get access.

There are the odd letters and notes found – a fax I sent to D when I was marooned at the Adelaide Writers Festival, sharing a session with Arundhati Roy (cold, snobbish), and feeling lonely: 'the only one I want is you'. Or the card I gave my mother when I nervously brought out my first novel: 'To my mother/from whom I came/I wasn't what she probably/expected/but/I've always known/I walked this earth/dressed in the garment of her love.'

There's a whole professional history there – different drafts of *Desperate Remedies* and *A Death in the Family*, as well as notes on a film group back in 1985 when we were fighting for short film to get funding recognition from the Film Commission.

A lot goes into the bin – duplicates, stuff no longer relevant. Joyfully, all my tax details from a much earlier time. Those dead, dead cheque books like vanquished tongues.

I always knew I'd have to start gleaning things, reducing, sending things away, apportioning among archives and sorting out what is strictly personal or autobiographical. Will I be like Walter Nash who kept every bus ticket? What might a future biographer want to know, even assuming such a person were to exist? The letter forgotten between the pages of something entirely boring? I have tended to be very openly autobiographical most of my life, so there will be very few surprises. And perhaps in some senses these very postings are my own act of letting go – a personal auto da fé whereby I lose my sensibilities to do with what is best kept private, indecently or decently withheld. Letting go for me is a very relaxing business, partly because I have resisted it so much all my life. But now is the time for cleansing, sorting, throwing away – and shuffling the essentials into the 'keep' pile. This will go on for days and weeks, maybe all year, the piles reducing according to a new form of logic which will emerge as I attempt to tidy my life away so I can make, or at least attempt to make, a reasonably clean exit.

February 23, 7.13 a.m.

We had a leg of lamb over the weekend and it was my role to sharpen the carving knife. Sharpening the carving knife – the sound of it, the action of it – sent an echo shivering through my body that was virtually physical – a small vibration of memory, welcome and rhythmic. I became my father. And my father was kind and good.

I have never really written about my rapprochement with my father, Gordon.

There's an almost fairy-tale symmetry to it: a kind father in childhood who was alienated by my gayness as I grew up, a bitter period of almost brutal alienation, followed by a very brief sweet farewell. It only occurred to me today there is another symmetry. Dad was dying of cancer of the throat. Some of the most important moments of rapprochement occurred in the cancer ward at Auckland Hospital.

This is what happened. I had driven Dad to hospital for radiation treatment. This in itself was surprising. I imagine my mother was playing bridge or caught in one of those internecine battles in which to lose a hand or a game meant a whole season went out of joint. Russell, my brother, was too busy being busy at that time in his life.

So it was me who drove Dad to the hospital that day. He was already desperately sick. His golfing clothes hung on him – slacks savagely belted together to a notch hitherto never reached, the Aertex shirt open at the stringy neck, the Hush Puppies seemingly too big for his toes – these pieces of theatrical masculinity supported him more than the bones of his body.

I drove his beautifully polished emerald-green Datsun, each seat lavishly covered in sheep skin. This car was his territory alone, almost a fetish object: it had nothing to do with my mother and her money (and her power). It was his frigate. He had handed over the keys. There was something casually ritualistic about this, unspoken in the urgency of the situation. He was sick, he was cowed with pain.

I hate to see people suffer. In that instant I forgave him everything, or almost everything. His abject state asked it, demanded it.

So here he was, riding into hospital in his Datsun, with his second son. Peter.

His once-pansy son, the boy he loathed, or at least the boy whose sexuality he loathed.

Oh, the arguments we had when I was in my twenties and coming out. How we yelled at one another, right into each other's faces. But as we got older, both of us, we began to suspect there were two different humans behind the political positions we took.

Maybe it was in one of these strange abeyances – a laying-down of arms – that it occurred to me to say, Yes, I was free that day. What was I doing anyway? Recovering from the suppurating wound of GOFTA, trying to get my career back on track?

We drove, I remember, through the Domain, from the Parnell side of town. It was in that long curved road which passes by the front of the Museum. I don't know why I am being so geographically specific: but it was there where a small miracle occurred. Dad looked at me with love. It was such a shock, such a mortifying moment, I didn't know how to react. Mortifying in that it required so little to crack open his heart. The smallest gesture. I could see where he was coming from: the utter surprise that at the end of his life, when he was scorned by his wife, scorned by his elder son (I'll get to that), it was me who had made myself available to help him.

We wound each other without thinking – or rather, the not thinking is what wounds. Bess could brusquely not make herself available to drive her dying husband to hospital (she was so close to him she didn't see he was dying). Russell had a high-powered career, he could not afford the time. (He was haunted, as it turned out, by the shade of his own death with AIDS. He could feel it coming.)

So it was left to me, the second son, third in the pecking order, to drive Dad to hospital. That was what was behind his look of love. A sense of incredulity that of all his family, it was me who was there.

We went inside the hospital, into what in memory stands as a dark low room. The people we were dealing with were young and brusque. I felt scandalised by their lack of respect. Dad was marked up – this is my memory – there were fluorescent lights on his naked chest. He lay there silent as an animal in a veterinary clinic. He was blasted. His thin gnarled old body, a presentiment of mine now.

It was then I found myself saying that this had to stop, this radiation. I was taken into another room. He was clearly dying, I said. He should be left alone to die in peace and comfort. It seemed to cause a stir. Who was I? Where did I fit in? I was angry. Probably I was angry about Dad dying but, more truthfully, the unresolved mess of our family life. Only unwillingly was it accepted that the radiation would end.

Dad went into hospital at this point. He died pretty much the night after. None of us was there. None of us knew he was so near to dying. He died quietly, capably, withdrawn into himself like a flower back into the bud from whence he came.

I went to see him, to make my peace. I was alone. I can't think where my mother was. Or brother. It seemed to have devolved to me to represent a family that was at odds with itself. My mother who had lived with my father with such animosity over so many years – 40 years – collapsed almost immediately. Russell was dead within a year. Mum fell apart like a building which has had an indispensable prop removed. Without any of us being aware of it this was the beginning of

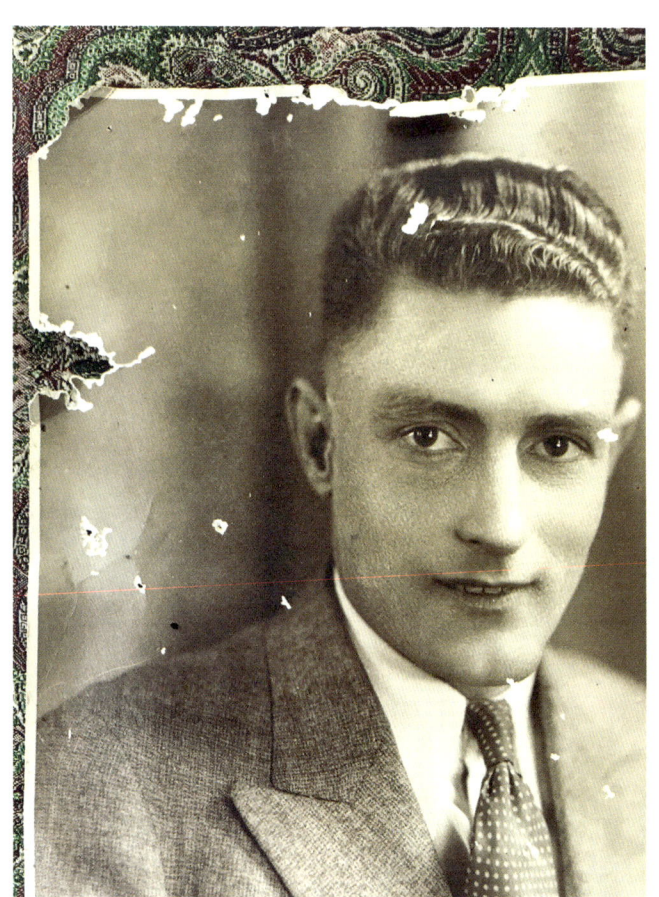

the dismantling – the whole family at this point would begin its slow-motion collapse.

So when people ask about the rapprochement it was this small, this slim – these few seconds on a ride into hospital when Dad turned to me and showed the shyness of his love.

February 24, 3.45 a.m.

It's a long time since I've been blissfully drunk. I don't drink much at all now because of my medical condition. But a few nights ago I had what is called a good drunk and it reminded me of the marvellously exultant mood that goes with drinking at its best. I'd forgotten the beautiful clear clarion call of a good drunk, a pellucid sense of seeing right to the heart of matter and, if surrounded by compatible companions, a wonderful sense of company, all of us virtually joining in a choral symphony, each person contributing their own special note.

Oh how I loved to drink in my youth. Like all nascent alcoholics there was an immediate sense of homecoming on the very first taste of alcohol – a shandy (red wine with water) in our kitchen at Pt Chev when I was just growing out of a kid. I didn't take to drink, though. I was frightened of what it unleashed in my parents who were of the hard-drinking postwar generation – that group of people who never funda-mentally adjusted to the disappointment of peace and the mild gruel that was postwar life. I hated what alcohol did to them. It's not like they were drunks – heavens, no. But it unleashed their secret bitterness, the snarling discontent of people living lives that didn't feel like their own. Dad became an alcoholic in the way of so many returned servicemen who used alcohol to cope with PTSD. This was so common nobody ever questioned it. Sozzled ex-servicemen were like the sky or bad weather. They just were.

So for a long time I avoided alcohol. But once I hit my twenties and met the Elam crowd, who all used alcohol as a way to levitate, I reconnected with my love affair with alcohol. Dubonnet when I was trying to be sophisticated. Martinis which were so strong on a virgin stomach I vomited. But alcohol and I moved into a lovely proximity, and my parents could relax now because when I came home I could have a 'spot' with them. I lost my prudish horror of alcohol.

But as everyone knows, alcohol is not a static liquid – it quickly extends to eat your whole life if you let it. I didn't. I was too much of a control freak for that, but god how I loved those breakouts into a really good drunk. There's really nothing like it because at its best it's companionable – a good drunk could never be done alone. It's back to that choral symphony I talked about earlier. It's inherently cheerful (or the melancholy is more deeply hidden) – I recognise one draws power from the other. You become prismatically brilliant as things formulate themselves with special sharpness. People say unallowable things. You slip the leash that society places on you in everyday life. You laugh a lot. Your body relaxes, and somehow the air whistles up from your stomach to your wind pipe and out of your mouth. Oh yes, you get wild all right, wonderfully wild. Then you need more alcohol to maintain that blistering brilliance. Besides, behind you is a history of hurt, of secret disappointments so painful you could never articulate them. You awaken at 3 a.m. haunted by them – things you wish you hadn't done, can't undo. But in that moment of brilliant drunkenness you feel you have worked out a way round that intractable problem. It's even better than that. You just forget all about it. You park it for a few glorious hours and run off on this escapade in which you are a brilliant and witty seer, immune to failure and especially immune to the ordinary inconvenience of a hangover. What does a mere hangover matter when you're having a riveting good time? Besides, aren't you owed a good time after all the shit you've lived through?

And so it all goes on, the unbeautiful bullshit, the untidy self-deceit, the unsettling feeling you've forgotten something or left something behind – some almost unknown self, an earlier self perhaps. Not more innocent, because you don't believe in that shit, but a self at the crossroads, just at that moment of uncertainty about which direction to take. Then you launch off anyway, as indecision is its own decision. And suddenly your life which once lay ahead of you is behind you and you're looking back at it and you're no longer drunk and you wonder . . . you wonder how or even why did it happen that way?

But a good drunk slam dunks all that. Trounces the indecision, delivers you back like a World War One combatant magically returned to the state you were in, on the day war was declared. You're complete again, unwounded, perfectly yourself.

It's a delusion, of course, but a beautiful one. (Oh stay with me a little longer please. Let me bathe in that wonderful and rare sense of completeness.) But that's the thing. You can't. It's a one-off. Or else you spend the rest of your life trying to get back into that peerless state. You become a boring old ordinary drunk, a one-star alcoholic.

So this little screed is just a salute to a wonderful night among friends, enjoying the rarest luxury for this old medical wreck – a beautiful drunk, a one-off as rare as a blue moon.

This is my parents' dinner service. It is astonishingly complete, right down to egg cups. It used to sit in a cupboard in the kitchen, glinting away behind glass. It was used at Christmas time and when we had guests. Then, as we all aged, it was used a bit more casually until finally, by the time my mother was in her nineties, we used it every time I came home for a meal. It was pleasing to use – it reminded us of the past, and its faint sense of ceremony was soothing. Then once I was dividing up my mother's house again, some instinct made me keep it, even though it was large and cumbersome. Other things I sent away – one of the most difficult things being the cutlery box in which we used to put the silver away every evening, having hand-dried it. The way the forks went into a special place, and knives, reminded me somehow of the formality of the family – how we all belonged in a particular place. It was a wedding present.

How I longed to keep that cutlery set. Off to the auction-eers it went. But somehow this dinner set survived, hidden away in a big old wooden box. I imagined I might give it to a cousin, but then I thought it might be an encumbrance. Finally D brought it up to Auckland to be auctioned. By such slim threads do we attach ourselves to the past.

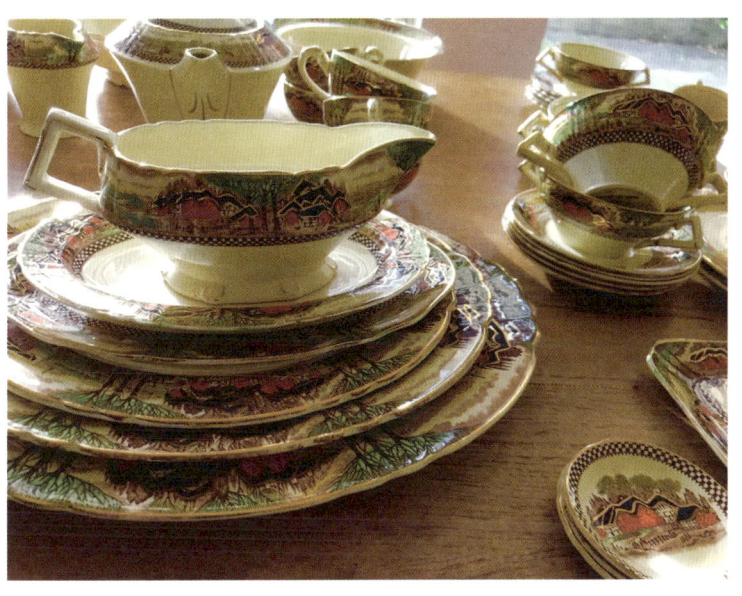

For me the gold lavished on an imaginary English village scene is part of the promise of my parents' marriage: it's what they hoped it would all be – dinner parties and candlelight and success. As it turns out, it's an archaic set of china which is now completely out of fashion. Nobody dreams any longer of England's green green lawns. It goes off to the auctioneer soon and with a bit of luck I won't know what happens to it.

February 28, 4.27 a.m.

Is there such a thing as cancer euphoria? There was apparently such a thing as TB euphoria. It was one of the things which powered Katherine Mansfield's tremulous, poignant writings towards the end of her life. I understand the mood. Everything appears almost unbearably precious. You're too happy, to the point of it being painful. Everything around you appears beautiful (more than possible, at this late summer into autumn season). But I've never heard of cancer euphoria. Cancer as a word is ugly, black in colour, bleak and lacking light. It is not associated with lyricism. And I cannot think offhand of any writer suffering cancer who has written significantly about it (though I could well be wrong here – I have not studied the field). I mean outside of 'cancer diaries', a title I find – how can I say this – loathsome? I myself am said to be writing 'a cancer diary', despite my saying that the title made me vomit. I hated the idea. Why? Because all of life is reduced to one plaint. I am more than my cancer, I hope. In fact, if these postings have had any subliminal message it is that I have a life so much more wide-ranging than this one terrible disease. Yet I am my disease too. I am its mortality. And there seems no easy way round a quick definition: 'A diary of a literary gent, an almost-famous homo, lover of cats and decor who incidentally has a terminal disease which preoccupies him day by day, hour by hour'. I saw Simon Wilson's cancer diary in the *Herald* on Saturday, felt sorry to hear that he too has this fucking stupid disease. I sped-read his piece and marvelled at the difference between men, authors, people (of course).

Simon is a wonderful writer, undoubtedly one of the best journalists in New Zealand. His writing is always limpid, highly intelligent, and he manages to make complex situations comprehensible which, god knows, is a great gift. His approach to his diagnosis is less emotional than mine, more fact-based, more transactional, you might say. On the same day, there was Stephen Fry, doing a public outing of the fact he also has prostate cancer. This was an excruciating live-to-camera performance which I don't doubt he already bitterly regrets. There's no transition here between wit and something which does not require the cosmetics of wit, only clarity. How do we speak? How do we say what we have to say?

It's not easy, yet the struggle itself is energising. I want to write around it – cancer; I want to write about anything that interests me really. Of course I keep coming back to the implacable fact – the wall I can't help but bang into. There's also the daily struggle through ailments. Like today – now this is unglamorous – when my reaction to chemo seems to be unstoppable diarrhoea. I'm lucky. I could have nausea, which I regard as much worse. But am I more than my symptoms? Am I more than my diagnosis? Or can I write my way through it? I am almost pathetically dependent on writing – and to be even more specific – writing here, making these posts. It's here where I try and make sense of my situation. It's here where I really exist as much as in my physical body. So is this a cancer diary? I suppose it is, for lack of a better term. But my wish is that it is more than this. It's not about chronicling my death so much as my urge for life.

I wonder if all of us were given, say, five to ten years to live whether it wouldn't help many of us find definition, closure, clarity, purpose even. I wonder.

March 1, 3.27 a.m.

Every civilised man needs a good woman friend. My great friend for the past 25 years has been the distinguished writer, Shonagh Koea. We clicked when we met at, of all things, a wedding. (I say this because weddings seem like the picking fields of her novels.) I had read her latest novel, a marvellously fruity affair called *Staying Home and Being Rotten* (her titles are always small masterpieces. *Yet Another Ghastly Christmas* is from her oeuvre.) Nobody was writing like Shonagh in New Zealand at the time. She was witty and highly observant of the foibles of everyday life. Shonagh herself was distinctive, with thick black hair and the sardonically amused look of a Roman emperor or empress who had come to live among ordinary folks and come to accept their mistakes. It turned out she grew up in Hawke's Bay, so we had a mythos to share.

I am unsure now how we came to write letters to one another. But very quickly we were writing letters each week,

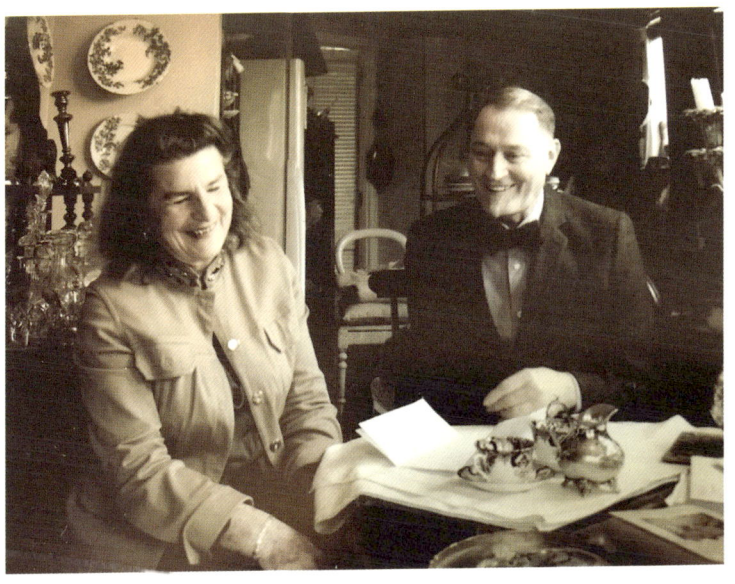

even if we were in the same city. There was a lot to comment on: literary parties attended with the usual rash of bad behaviour; ordinary aperçus about daily living; writerly problems – Shonagh was far ahead of me as a novelist, and her letters were like an informal guidebook to her highly idiosyncratic methods of composition. Shonagh, it turned out, also had a great streak of kindness, and she was very kind to me when I trudged through some seemingly impenetrable crisis or other. She had the advantage of being slightly older than me and her wisdom was accrued from a life not only well lived but tried at times by great difficulties. We laughed a lot. And we also had an abiding love of cats – the silence of cats, the companionship of cats, the wisdom of cats. When our respective cats died we mourned not together, because Shonagh is not that type of person – but we shared an empathy of grief. She understood pain both human and animal. With my cancer she has been astute, endlessly patient and deeply understanding. I only ever had one sibling and he died long, long ago now. Shonagh is by way of a sibling I never had.

But now we arrive at what seems a problem. I have safely within a box in the watertight back shed not hundreds but thousands of letters from Shonagh (just as she has thousands of letters from me). D when he is being amusing says he plans to live off the income of the edited letters of PW and SK.

In fact we have both informally agreed that the letters go to an archive of our choice.

So there is no problem. It is just the sheer sprawling vastness of the correspondence which seems daunting. (52 weeks a year, at least a letter a week, times 25 years = 1300.) What faux pas, too, have I committed to print (or handwriting)? A good bit of literary gossip is sprinkled through the letters, often mediated by the kindness of Tiberius as he nudges a slave off the cliff at Capri. How will I appear in the mirror of my prose? It's a risky business, saving letters, as they tend to backfire – look at Philip Larkin and his frightful letters to his secretary Monica Jones. One can always specify the letters are to be consulted only. And there's always the possibility of a 25-year ban on anyone looking at the letters. That can seem a bit forbidding, but a cooling-off period is not necessarily that bad. I don't want people to think these letters are a hotbed of gossip and mischief. As Shonagh often replied when people asked, 'What do you and Peter talk about?': 'The price of onions.'

Every civilised man needs a close woman friend. Shonagh Koea, with her marvellous treasure trove of letters, has been mine.

March 2, 4.26 a.m.

There is nothing more exhausting than looking after someone long term. I know this from looking after my mother. But then I didn't look after her on a daily, hourly basis – this amounts to a scrutiny of the soul which is so eviscerating you become worn away to little more than a shadow. Bess lived in a Ryman's retirement village, in studio accommodation, for the last ten years of her life. On the whole, within the confines of a system which is industrialised caring of the aged, she experienced good care. This was entirely due to the staff – by which I mean nurses and those women who replaced her towels or cleaned her bathroom, most of whom were unfailingly good humoured and humane. This meant I never really experienced the burden of looking after her personally. Or rather those few times I did, it was in a crisis situation which was so stressful I felt as if I were going insane.

Yet just being 'a good son', with all this implies in terms of attention, affection and supervisory care (intervening sometimes to ensure her care was correct for her needs), was curiously exhausting in the long run. You might think a 100-year-old would be frail and sickly – well, Bess was certainly frail, but she had a life force which was phenomenal. I was the sickly one compared to her resonant love of life. But I gradually came to know the exhaustion involved in keeping someone alive. It is not a life-support system per se but something more diffuse – perhaps lending your life energy to them. Listening, paying attention, being kind, turning up regularly. So while I did not care for her on a daily basis I did care for her in a larger sense. And because I loved her as a mother and also a curiosity – I was biologically linked to a woman almost entirely different in her tastes from me, who did not read, who regarded intellectual virtues as a vague and impenetrable mystery, who adored sport – yet I felt almost a sense of terror when she neared death (only for her to repeatedly recover). I was driven to exhaustion by her thirst for life – in the end by her refusal to die. So I did know the depth of exhaustion involved in looking after someone.

But recently I have had to change my specs. For no particular reason D had started to feel weak, directionless, lacking enjoyment in everyday things. To me it seemed inexplicable, worrying. Then I had a sudden perception: he was exhausted by the long-term task of looking after me. It had been going on now for five long months. We had moved beyond the excitement of crisis and the terror of the diagnosis. We had clung together tremulously, barely able to breathe when it was all happening. Miraculously he never faltered.

Without my ever asking, he took on the burden of looking after me. He began cooking, which was something I had always enjoyed doing. More than this he began to cook really beautiful vegetarian meals. It took me a long time to work out this was in response to his understanding of the role of overconsumption of meat in relation to cancer. I had just thought it was part of a personal predilection. (The blindness of a partner – too close to actually see.)

Suddenly I saw I was exhausting him just as my mother had exhausted me. I understood too something deeper about this state of exhaustion, because I myself had been through it. You are caught in this eternally incomplete state whereby you want the person to stay alive, you want them to stay well, you want to go on loving them, but you also subconsciously know the only relief you are ever going to get is when they die: this marks the finite point of the endless tension. But this in itself is shocking. So you are caught in between two powerful emotions, one apparent, one barely glimpsed. I am not saying of course that D is waiting for me to die. That would be grotesque. But from my own experience with my mother, I understood the conflicted emotions involved in looking after someone in a terminal condition (as in fact extreme old age is). You had to keep going, you had to keep being cheerful, or at least not depressed. You had to provide support, the nourishment of love: but what about you, the essence of you? Was that being fed, allowed to live, allowed to feel free? In that lies the great problem of these situations.

One is bound together by love: death, to a degree, is the

solution but also – and this is what is so painful – it is the very thing you dread, the very thing that will end what is both a beautiful companionship and a duty so harsh it almost kills you. How to balance the two so that one does not eat away at the other? How to stay alive with all your emotions intact?

Now it was my turn to nourish, to look at him carefully in silence and try and work out what was best to do so we both flourish, one supporting the other.

March 4, 5.27 a.m.

'You look so well!' I'm so often greeted with these words. It's my low-level paranoia which dictates an accusation in the words. Shouldn't I be 'looking sick', whatever that means? Pale, hobbling, visibly in decline? Am I some kind of fraud, milking the sympathy of the public while secretly being quite healthy? The fact is I continue to look surprisingly well – most days. I still have wisps of hair after my third chemo. But this isn't the full story. There is a behind-the-scenes reality which is less roseate. This is the one D is privy to, when I awaken full of aches and feeling incoherent – hardly a whole person. I only need to forget my pills once for my body to react with a vengeance. It's frightening, my dependence on long-release morphine. I revert very quickly to the state I was in when it all began. So the bone pain is always just hovering there, awaiting its moment to force an entrance. I'm not complaining, just commenting on my reality. I actually look completely different when I am home alone, feeling lousy. I do 'look sick'.

After my third chemo I seemed to suffer from a deep tiredness. So deep I could barely summon up the energy to move from one room to another. I also had thrush really badly in my mouth – so demoralising when you can't speak or eat, two of my favourite activities. So this is the obverse of my 'looking so well' in public. It's an act – but a very good act.

March 6, 2.43 a.m.

For whatever reason, D has suddenly started to plan ahead. This is a complete mood swing (he's as subject to them as I am). There's huge gusto in his plans. Bathroom renovations. A tree to be cut down and the garden replanned. The list is long and detailed. I'm full of admiration for this new energy level – at the same time understanding why he wants to escape the frustrating stalling of the present. It's kind of like a hurdling over all this waiting and sitting round and hurtling into a future which – theoretically – I'll also share. Or isn't just the planning excitement enough in itself? Otherwise we are left here in the present, watching everything so cautiously, made timid by the intervention of chance – a rash, a swollen foot, thrush in the mouth. So much of my experience of this 'sickness' is predicated on how you see it, on the view you take of it. I try and position myself in terms of longevity, but another way to look at it is: you have so little control over what's happening to you that there's just a tiny area of manoeuvre – and this is where will comes into it, the will to live, to survive, to surmount if humanly possible – and you have to try and expand that area so it becomes representative of you as a human. To plan a future you may not occupy isn't completely stupid. It has elements of fantasy, yes – even enjoyable fantasy. (Doesn't the bus driver, exhausted by the routine of his job, dream of a holiday on the East Cape?) But for me it carries some elements of sadness. I ask myself, Will I be here to enjoy it? But this is precisely the wrong question to ask: it's looking in the wrong direction. The right direction is to enjoy the hustle of the planning, the activity, the hyperactivity of choosing this over that; and in this way one moves round the immutable area where one has so little choice it amounts to almost no choice. So this species of movement, frantic, energetic, joy-filled, becomes my occupation – D's preoccupation. We plan movement to escape stasis. That seems about right from where I stand now.

March 7, 2.32 a.m.

Solitude. What a wonderful word. D and I have been together every day and night since I got sick five long months ago (barring the nights I spent in hospital). We have grown into each other like two trees with our boughs interwoven. But it isn't without its strains, since we are – or rather were – two independent men. Before I got sick – now that is an historic phrase – I often spent quite long times apart from D. We both had separate careers. That was how our relationship worked. But then I got sick and my independence evaporated and my dependence grew. It became a relationship of almost overpowering intimacy. So tonight when D steps on a plane to go away to Auckland to work for three days is the first time I have . . . wriggled my toes and walked about the house aimlessly, feeling the in-tide of solitude. (Just as he will be looking forward to time away.)

The one thing I am most looking forward to is sleeping during the day uninterrupted. With nobody in the house there is no distant footstep or door closing – nothing to interrupt that sinking into sleep wherein all things begin to be marvellously rearranged in your head.

Solitude. Such a beautiful word. I aim to do nothing for three days. I aim to have no appointments, no commitments.

(Hopefully I won't catch anything, fall ill. These three days are the days when my immunity is at its very lowest.)

March 8, 3.34 a.m.

I hadn't counted getting – I'm sorry – diarrhoea during the night. (Diarrhoea is one of the side effects of the type of chemo-therapy I'm on.) It's a kind of covert attack that suddenly becomes alarmingly real. I realised D had talked of us needing to get toilet paper – there was some but an alarmingly small amount. It was in the zone of 1.30 a.m. – I was still trying to maintain the 'I'm still asleep, I'm just doing this stuff, then I'll drop back into bed again and go to sleep.' But once I was heading back to bed my rational mind awoke and said, 'You have to take two tablets as prescribed by the oncologist.' I knew the drill. I went to my study and got the little green and fawn fuckers. Really. They're so efficient but so toxic when added to all my other pills. Anyway, by that time I'm awake.

Back to bed. One more alarm during the night, just to perfectly jag me out of a deep sleep pattern.

I awoke late, in a scramble, had my breakfast – actually not my normal breakfast at all, just toast and tea which showed how disturbed my pattern was – had my pills, showered and went off to have my coffee. At the last moment before going out the door I glanced at the mirror and saw, to my horror, my hair was standing on end like a lunatic's. I realised it was going to be one of those days. Scrambled. Out of sync. Not working properly. Outside my skin.

Only gradually during the day did I manage to calm down. I even slept for two hours, then I began to succumb to this enormous backlog of sleepiness, as if I simply couldn't get enough. In between I read that marvellous novel, Olivia Manning's *The Great Fortune*, published in 1960, about a flaky British couple in Budapest as the Nazis close in.

But then I dropped back into sleep again. When I awoke, I decided on some green medicine which really didn't help the sleepiness. I missed D with an absolute need as if he were a drug being withdrawn from my system. I texted him but he was busy at work. Gradually I came to understand I had to organise my time, get real with being on my own. I started sorting my papers, threw a whole lot out, then later considered that I was actually throwing out just what might be of interest to that entirely theoretical researcher in the future, the 'good traveller' who might come my way. (I accept this may never happen. But like a good host one should be prepared.) The day passed, and I cooked myself a delightful dinner with Peg the cat following each movement of the lamb on my fork to my mouth with much scrutiny. It was nearing the end of my second day of lowest immunity.

Much much later at night D and I spoke on the phone. How I loved to hear the timbre of his voice. It was like stroking the fur of a cat. Then I surprised myself by saying to him, after we had said our goodbyes, in a quick lullaby, *I love you I love you I love you.* He laughed in surprise and said I love you too. I went to sleep slipping down the slope into a honey of sweetness and happiness. We had spoken to one another.

March 12, 6.03 a.m.

Preparing. Limbering up. You write a book and you live in the forest of words. You can't see beyond it and everything within it is gigantic, important and significant. Finally you deliver the book – you walk out of the forest and with almost astonishing speed it's a long way behind you. Besides, there's all that suppressed living that you couldn't do when you lived in the forest. Now you set out to enjoy yourself – you almost set out to forget the book. Then – and I'm at the 'then' stage – the book looms back into view. You're going to have to speak about it, read from it, be a specialist in it. But – and this is me – you have this moment of paranoia that you've forgotten everything to do with it. You can't remember a thing. You doubt very much you wrote it. But this is even worse – you're going to have to sit a test on it. And Kim Hill is going to be the examiner. Will she ask such difficult questions that I won't know how to answer them? Or is this a 3 a.m. screaming nightmare? After all, Kim Hill is the best interviewer of writers, hands down.

So I'm in the process of reacquainting myself with *Dear Oliver* after a long period in which I simply let it go. It's not like

I'm exactly swotting but I'm back to being friendly with the book, its contents and what I spent so much energy struggling to articulate. I've got to be clear on what drove me to write the book, as well as its intricacies and pleasures. I'll get there. That book is my best friend at the moment.

Not only this. I'm walking. I'm practising walking. I've been so energy-less for such a long time, I've got out of the way of walking any distance. So I'm limbering up. I'm getting ready.

March 14, 2.04 a.m.

I listened to my interview with Kim Hill this morning on Replay Radio and was heartened that I didn't make a complete fool of myself. She seemed in a positively jolly mood, and I said 'Yes yes yes' much too often. I found it odd being treated as a terminal case, as someone, in the longer or shorter term, dying, as this is not the way I conceptualise my life. (How do I conceptualise it? With as little space between me living in a daily sense and the bigger question of when/how will I die – so little space this huge question does not exist.)

Then this afternoon I bumped down to an interview with a local journalist for a free newspaper.

'But do you make a living?' I wonder how many visiting architects, lawyers, even sportsmen and women are ever asked this question. Yet at a certain level of journalism it is de rigueur to ask the visiting writer. I call it the revenge of the journalist-who-once-dreamt-of-being a writer. You may be talking to someone who hasn't 'had time to read your book' but they hold the upper hand as they run through the checklist which goes from 'Did you always want to write?' to 'Which is your favourite book?' before swinging off into 'Have any of your books sold well?' This, again, is from the journalist who hasn't actually read the book. It's a species of low-level humiliation, whereby the lack of intellectual vitality of the community is revealed by a deficiency of interest in the journalist. 'This is just another job' seems to hover just beyond the perimeter of his questions. Of course, since he has not read the book – he has barely read the press pack – he can't ask any questions about it. 'What's the press reaction to the book been then?' was a further crafty question meant to reduce the author to a quivering mess. 'Well, it went on the bookshelves yesterday . . .'

And so it went on, a press interview in an undisclosed town somewhere in the North Island . . .

Later I went for a walk by the sea which, post storm, had the most magnificent waves. I stood there a long while and looked at the waves. Gradually I felt myself again.

March 15, 1.49 a.m.

Yesterday I was down in the pits after the non-interview by the journalist-who-had-not-read-the book. Then today a friend meeting me for coffee said had I seen Wardini's window? There's a whole window display, she said. After coffee, we whizzed along to look and I was astonished, delighted, touched to see a whole window display featuring the book and the launch in Napier.

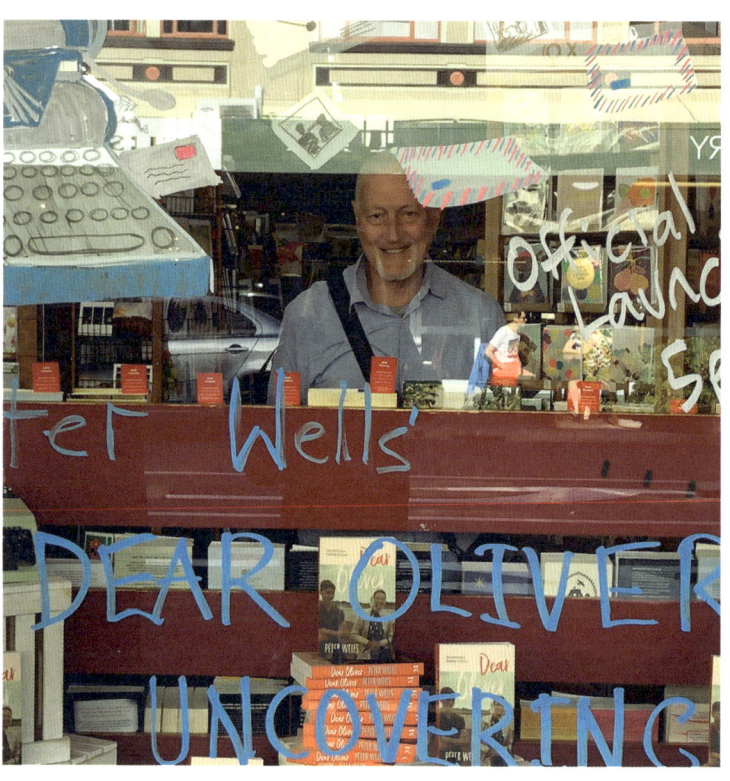

Immediately my mood changed to delight. (This is my friend, Annie's, photo.) Is this the nature of a book launch, I wonder: a kind of manic kaleidoscope of moods going from bleak despair through to unrealistic celebration? Where's the medium line? And will I be able to speak well? With my cancer I've developed this utterly weird echo in my chest which sounds like cellophane paper crinkling. It certainly lends an invalid flourish (which I do not want). I'm all over the place mood-wise. But I have to say crossing the road and finding this utterly delightful, inventive display lifted my spirits enormously. As the photo shows. #chuffed

March 19, 1.52 p.m.

On a visit to Wellington I had time for a catch-up with Georgina Beyer who I have known since she appeared in *Jewel's Darl* in 1987, a friendship that went on through her years as a politician and the celebrity of being the first trans MP in the world; through *Georgie Girl*, the doco that Annie Goldson and I co-directed, which recorded some of the dilemmas of that time; and onwards till now when we are both experiencing health challenges. Georgie got a new kidney last year and is settling into that. We had a lot to talk and reminisce about, but also in a way to celebrate – a good long friendship with something almost shy at its heart, a concern for the other person even though our lives are very different. We asked the waitress to take our photo and here we are, two people getting on in years but determined to enjoy the sunshine and the experience of an enriching friendship.

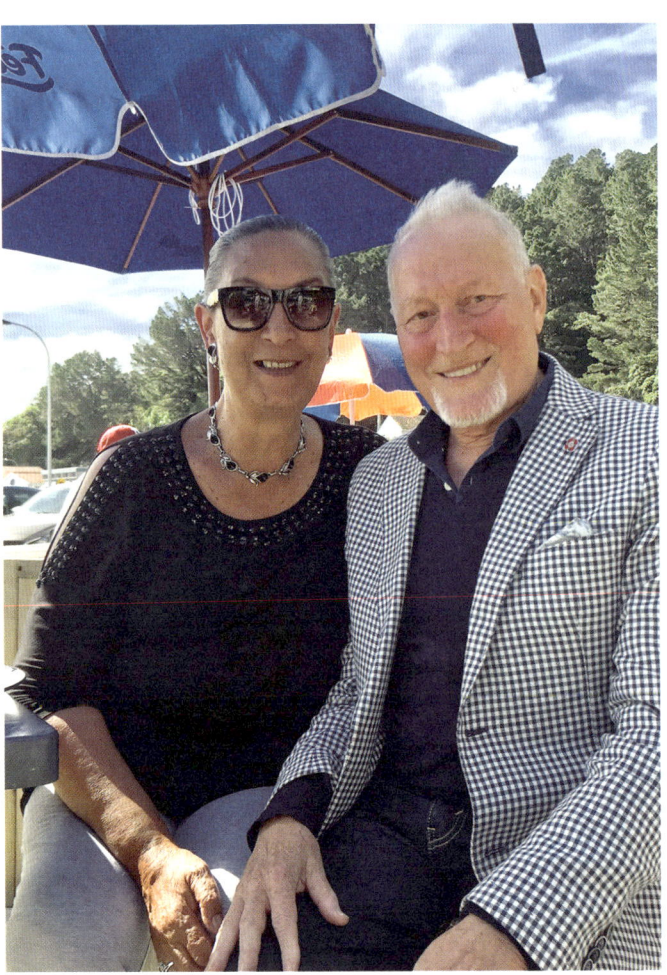

March 20, 12.40 p.m.

Tomorrow's my book launch and today I feel like shit. I'm back to the 'stomach upset' blues, a particularly levelling complaint. I end up feeling weak and dirty as old dishwater. Tomorrow, too, I'm having a CT scan – that's how my launch day begins. I have to fast from 8.30 a.m. to have the scan at 10 a.m. This was one of the very early scans I had, 'when it all began'. It won't be as frightening – I'm an old hand now. But my mood's still all over the place.

It doesn't help that I saw on FB that David Colquhoun has died in Masterton Hospital. I knew him primarily from the Alexander Turnbull Library. It was he you dealt with when selling manuscripts. He was a lean sprinter of a man, slightly nervous – but this was about doing the right quintessential thing. I hesitate to say it, as it is no longer regarded as a quality, but 'he was a gentleman' – intelligent, fair and sensitive. I also had a much more personal connection. During the Springbok tour, during the Hamilton game, I was outside the stadium with friends. We managed to pull down a wire fence and then we all ran towards the stadium. I was a fast runner and got to the parked trucks first. But as I looked down the chasm between trucks, I saw police with their truncheon-type weapons ready. I had so much momentum up I was poised to run into the chasm. But David, who I knew only by sight, grabbed hold of the back of my outfit and yanked me backwards. He saved me. This was such an instinctive but kind action. In the mêlée of the afternoon, I never thanked him. I thank him now.

I'm sorry for this melancholy undertow.

Today I'm flat tide out, but I hope by the early evening I'll be all right. I'll be back inside my skin. I've got my lines to run – the few pages from *Dear Oliver* I'll read at the launch tomorrow night. Pray god my voice does not wobble and I become emotional. I can already feel myself becoming a little better. Maybe just writing this here has cleared my throat, so to speak. I said on Kim Hill the extraordinary thing about posting on here was the feeling of being accompanied. Illness is so isolating. Writing here calms me and connects me and now I am no longer in my study on my own but in another world where other people exist . . . not so much hello darkness, as greetings to sunlight flittering away on the carpet . . . I can see the pattern on the carpet . . .

March 21, 12.56 a.m.

I did not expect to be on a CT scanning bed on the morning of my launch. Or to be more correct I had hurriedly agreed to the appointment without thinking through its emotional weight. (I was only in Auckland for a few days. It needed to be done. It was the first chance the oncologist had to see what my tumours were doing.) I was emotionally unprepared. I did all the right things – fasted from 8 o'clock, meaning I got up before daylight to have tea and porridge. I drove to Mercy Hospital only to find the familiar place I went to was CT MRI, not plain CT. Simple things like this tend to rock me. I went to the front of the building, registered, and was told I had to drink a large – a very large – amount of water. Then off into a cupboard to strip. There is something so levelling in taking all your clothes off, including rings and watch. 'You can keep your brief on,' the foreign-born nurse said to me. I went into the room where a doughnut-shaped machine was. So far so familiar. I was positioned – and this is the thing. This is when I stopped really being Peter Wells and became this thing to be positioned. A needle was introduced. An iodine solution was flushed through my veins by another nurse or technician. She kindly explained it would leave a metallic taste in my mouth and I might feel like I'm going to the toilet. Then she left the room. My thingness – the impossibility of being anything else but an invalid – was heightened as the bed advanced towards the doughnut ring, my arms raised and clasped (I liked to think) like a 13th-century Christ in a crucifixion scene – you have to think of something. I clasped my fingers together and I felt an infinite relief as my left fingers touched my right fingers as if I were asserting the primacy of my body – and then an American male voice barked 'Breathe in.' I breathed in and held my breath. 'Breathe!' the same voice barked. It was my natural inclination so I was pleased to obey. This happened twice. Suddenly and surprisingly quickly, it was all over.

Somehow defeated and a little soiled by experience, I went back to the cupboard to resume the appearance of being Peter Wells.

I got in the car and drove away – my mood still low, interrupted. I could not allow this. I drove to my favourite local cafe and ordered a latte and a raisin scone of the sort which is rough as scoria and dimpled all over by moist raisins. I thought to my manic self: Be careful on this day of days.

Last night I had the most wonderful book launch. Stephanie Johnson delivered a funny, apt launch speech, full of her genius for wit and touching truths, and after I said a few words I spent the rest of a very warm evening signing books. I was so busy I didn't take a single photo, I'm afraid.

Below are the few words I said before I did a reading:

This morning I had a CT scan and as I went into a room to undress I experienced that strange sense of how insubstantial a persona is. I was suddenly no longer Peter Wells, I was a vulnerable body, a human made a little anxious by what lay immediately ahead.

If I have learnt anything from the past six months it's both how vulnerable I am – and yet oddly enough – how strong I am. Sometimes you need to be separated from your persona for you to understand it, understand who you are.

Dear Oliver was written while my mother was alive, then, towards the end, as she lay dying. This profound experience – day into night – underlies the whole book, is the fundamental bridge over which the book passes.

But it's also written in the form of a letter to the future. The very title of the book is addressed to an eight-month-old baby to whom I try to explain the past of his Pākehā ancestors.

Bess my mother, by contrast, was 100 years old – a living example of a colonial ancestor. Born in 1916 she exemplified a pioneer past with some of its anxieties and some of its simple graces.

I had just finished the tough business of editing the book when I became ill, got my diagnosis and plunged headfirst into another reality. How pleased I was that I had the hard form of a nearly completed book on which to lean. This is a book I have wanted to write all my life – addressing my ancestors on my mother's side of the family, and indirectly addressing my mother herself.

Love, that thing which undoes us and yet makes us whole, that thing which causes more pain than anyone can bear yet also such intense pleasure nothing else equals it – love underlies this book. Love for my mother and love, in a different sense, for what I might call my motherland which is the hidden geography of this book. (Motherland in the sense of the stories she told about her family, but motherland too in the sense of something familiar, a homeland, somewhere where I belong.)

But I need to also address something else at the launching of this book. It is cushioned on some of the feelings aroused by my Facebook postings when I became ill, then The Spinoff rendition of 'Hello Darkness' which reached out to a wider audience still. Suddenly I seemed in digital contact with a wide range of people, many of whom connected with me on a very personal level (just as I had written very personally about my experiences with both mortality and illness).

Just today, when I posted about my grumpy sense of disavowal – of being stripped of my identity and returned to that of an invalid – a kind friend in Vancouver sent me a message: 'I think perhaps you are more loved at this time in your life than ever before. Your words reach deep. It is only human that others react with love back at you.' I replied, 'Oh goodness, what a truly lovely thought – like a golden raincoat?' and she replied, 'Yes to offset the showers.' I want to acknowledge this golden raincoat you have given me. If I was stripped of my identity to go into the CT machine, here I am awarded an invisible golden raincoat to withstand the metaphorical showers that we all have to endure. Thank you for your kindness, thank you for your aroha – and thank you for just being here.

March 24, 9:46 a.m.

D took this photo of me yesterday when I was in the deepest of sleeps, helped along again by dear old Peg who kept a paw on me for company. I spent yesterday thinking through all my impressions from the Wednesday book launch in Auckland, sorting them out as they all occurred in such a rush. Probably while sleeping I was sorting . . . and dreaming.

March 27, 2.49 p.m.

Some staggering news. Or as Steve Braunias put it, sudden, glorious news . . .

Can I cope with good news? I've inured myself by retaining a sense of hardy disbelief, by soldiering forth in a stony haze of obliviousness. What do I do when good news turns up? (I'm writing this in the chemotherapy room, which is more like a kitchen at a church hall during a women's parishioners meet – it's almost carelessly cheerful.) But today when I met with the oncologist she told me my CT scan had come back delivering the good news that my tumours had shrunk by half. She even

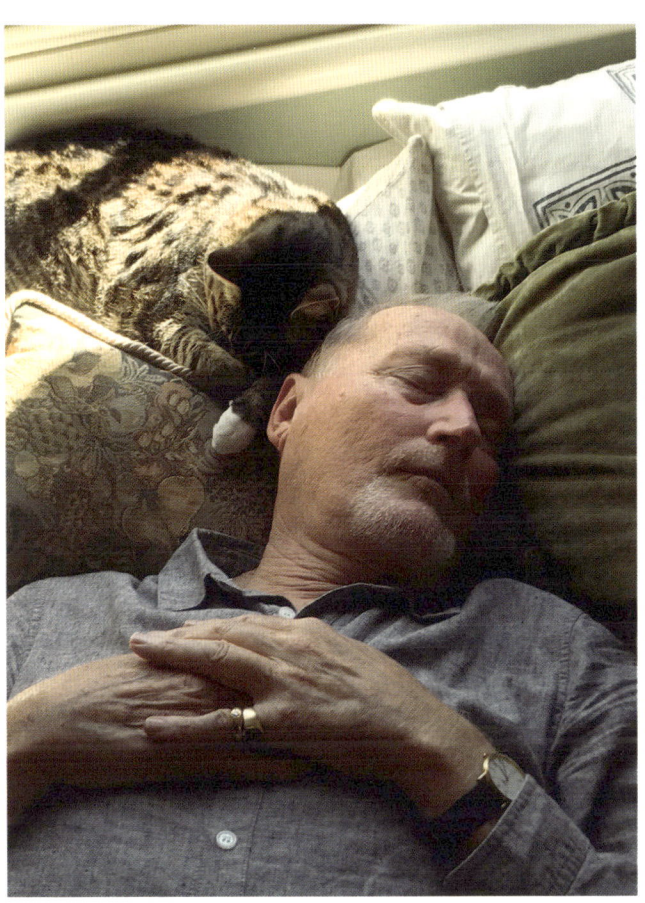

went so far as to describe the scan as 'beautiful'. Can a scan be beautiful? Certainly, when it delivers such stellar results.

I sat there stupefied, incapable of asking the meaning of this in terms of the bigger picture (why rain on my own parade?). I have been told so often I look so well (suspiciously well?) that now it can be confirmed that my cancer is not advancing at a fast pace but – maybe? – momentarily? – long term? – has lurched to a halt. Let's not ask now whether it is momentary or permanent. Let's not ask any of those drizzling questions but accept that, for this day now, this week now, my luck has held.

I still have another half hour in chemotherapy till I can get out. I won't run or jump or leap or cry. I'm too used to living with my condition for that. Besides, as always, nobody will answer the big question: how long have I got? Is it, in fact, a question that has an answer? Or is the scale more elastic than I had previously thought? Does one swallow make a summer? I don't know. I don't know. I don't know. That titanic life force that pervaded my mother's life has leapt into mine. I cannot stride but I can walk.

March 28, 4.45 a.m.

The waiting room is a place of many private moods. There is no cross-chat between people waiting. There is, however, discreet surveillance. This goes along the lines of: Which one has it (nearly everyone is in pairs) and how bad are you? Where do you fit on the trajectory of cancer? For example, yesterday there was a desperately thin young woman in a summery flute of a frock – she was so weak she had to be helped along. For someone like this we both gaze hungrily – so this is what it's like – but look away, as it is a heartbreaking spectacle.

The waiting room is always quiet, though there is innocuous pop music playing. There is art on the walls, up-to-date magazines (though as D pointed out, not the mag with the cover that said 'This is the only woman who made the Queen cry'). By such trivialities we divert ourselves. The receptionist is vague: she's too busy on the phone and does not recognise you, even though you have been coming there quite a few times.

We're all sitting waiting to see the oncologist who will determine our progress – or rather illuminate our progress or lack thereof. We're impatient, all of us, though we all mimic people who are busy reading magazines. Every so often a side door bursts open – these people have a different rule of silence – and it's someone from the chemotherapy room. This is a site of busyness, of activity, of doing. This is a place where bells ring and people come and go.

But we wait in silence.

Suddenly my oncologist appears outside her office door. She is smiling, but she is often smiling so I don't make much of this. She has to smile, sympathetically, through all sorts of failings, humiliations. But today, once we sit down and the door is closed – this closing of the door is always an important part of the ritual, as what we are to talk about can be painful – she appears positively rhapsodic. She quickly explains the wonderful news. I have trouble hearing for some reason. But I do hear 'tumours shrunken in half'. She talks further, illustrating the CT report, but I can't really comprehend the medical terminology though again I hear 'shrunken in size'.

This is related again and again. But somehow I am locked like a machine which can't quickly adapt. 'That's wonderful,' my lips say, and I turn to D and say, 'It's wonderful isn't it?' I'm dazed. The oncologist is so happy, she's a hay bale ablaze in summer sunlight, she's a circus turn at the highest height doing dazzling turns. But I am somehow slow to catch up.

She asks if I have any ongoing problems. Not really, apart from my usual reaction to chemo which is diarrhoea. She suggests I take medication for it in advance. But what does it mean? a voice says in my head. Am I going to live now? I don't dare ask this outrageously naked question. But what does it mean? I seem to be coming awake now. Will I live? Will I be alive for longer now, guaranteed? Or is nothing guaranteed? But I'm much too well bred – too timid – to ask this huge question.

We discover I only have two more chemotherapy sessions to go, not six. It's clear the session is over. Time is money. And I need to go in for my chemotherapy session now. We say our goodbyes. Yes, we all agree. It's wonderful news. Wonderful.

Only later, much later, does it occur to me the oncologist was so rhapsodically happy because how often did she have the chance to deliver good news? How much of her professional life was made up of mediating between terrible news and some slim hope – between possible improvements against devastating impossibilities? I had been obdurate in not joining in, in supplementing her very real burst of happiness. I had been slow and dazed, almost disbelieving. But for her it was a rare holiday in hope. She had a right to be so riotously happy. I see that now over my left shoulder as I advance into a new day, lighter, more buoyant. Yes, I am alone now. It is a day later. The news has sunk in. Yes, I can cry. And so, I am afraid,

I bawl on my own, only now realising the weight I've been living under.

Later:
I find I am walking round the house whistling. I realise I haven't whistled for a very long time. The only problem is – and what day doesn't have its problems – Ajax the cat keeps turning up, as whistling is my way of telling him his tucker is ready. Instead he gives me reproving looks: as in, are you insane or a fraud? Or both? I don't care. My whistling days have come back.

April 2, 5.27 a.m.

A kind friend said to me, 'You have been on such a high with the book launches and the news about your tumours, it's absolutely natural that you'd crash.' Now why couldn't I see that about myself, especially as I seem or pretend to specialise in being self-aware?

April 6, 3.24 p.m.

I heard today that 'Hello Darkness', The Spinoff edited version of these postings, is a finalist in the 2018 Voyager Media Awards. It's in the personal essay section. I'm pretty thrilled, as I had been sitting on my bed, googling life expectancy rates with Stage 4D prostate cancer. I realise this seems a hyper-morbid thing to be doing. But I go through these stages of trying to work out exactly what is happening. Am I in remission? Or am I . . .

April 12, 2.39 a.m.

'I'm back from the dead.' This thought struck me today, when I was sitting in the doctor's room, waiting. The thought actually 'struck me' with almost a physical force. I've somehow pulled myself back from the gulf, the edge, the precipice. This wasn't just my energy – it was chemotherapy, all the pills, radiation, and the careful judgement of my oncologist and Alison, my doctor. Get me. I'm already turning it into an Oscar acceptance speech. But hey! I'm back from the dead. That's how I feel. It may not be literally true. There will be complications. But inside myself, even outside myself, I've got this incredible joy and life force

So it's farewell to Freddie the walker and to my crutches. They are being sent back. I can walk all right without them now. I have a walking stick, my own silver and black walking stick, which I use when I need some extra support.

It's only by looking back I can see how far I've come. But get this: I am being discharged from the Hospice programme. They're getting rid of me. They visited me today and said I am too well now to be in the programme. I feel – well, I feel a little frightened to be so abandoned. Don't I really need them? Apparently my GP can recommend I go back onto the programme if need be. The truth is, I wasn't using them enough. So I'm ejected. I feel a lot of things. Pride that I am progressing so well. Fear that I might suddenly get bad again and then what will I do? I'm still fragile, I know that. I'm completely dependent on morphine and other medicines to get through the day. I'm weak after months of not being able to walk more than a block.

Who am I? Who am I apart from my disease? For a long time now prostate cancer has overwhelmed my personality, or rather I saw myself in relation to the disease – withstanding it, getting round it, living with the moods that relate to it. Who am I apart from my disease? I guess I'll find out.

April 13, 4.06 a.m.

Today I got something I'd normally think was kitsch – a card from the funeral people who did my mother's funeral. Amazingly Bess died one year ago today – a fact I had completely overlooked. (I'm like a signpost pointing into the future; I can almost not bear to look back into the past.) In some ways, too, it hardly seems possible that Bess died only one year ago, because so much has happened in the interim.

One of the curveball questions Kim Hill threw at me was: If you hadn't been spending so much time looking after your mother, you might have taken better care of yourself, i.e. recognised your cancer and got early treatment. I dismissed this out of hand. The nature of prostate cancer is that it is a silent disease. Unless you're tested for PSA, you don't know what's happening in there. This didn't happen for a multitude of reasons. But did I wear myself out looking after my mother?

Incontestably. The long slow weight of looking after someone hesitating before the point of death is devastating. And surely there is a silent statement in the fact that since 12 April 2017, Bess's death date, I fell so ill I almost died – so sick I too hesitated before the brink. The huge drama of this sickness overwhelmed my life. My mother sped into the distant past as if tugged away by a typhoon. I limped, hobbled, pulled myself along on a walker day by day. But Bess, kind Bess, did not fade away. If anything, she helped me by modelling how to go along the way with grace. And fortunately I had written most of *Dear Oliver*, so that the book, which in its own way is a homage to her, existed. I'm so pleased it exists, just as I'm moved by the fact readers are finding some kind of truth within it. To a degree, to each reader Bess comes alive again. She is not dead. If that seems kitsch, I apologise. But isn't one of the purposes of art – of writing – to make something that is inherently fleeting last?

One year later, and here am I sitting in my car in the rain, waiting to go into another oncology appointment. Why did I not remember that yesterday was the date of her death? Because I am ravenously living. I'm alive. I'm full of plans. I met a friend for coffee. I worked on a short piece of non-fiction. I picked D up at the airport. I met a lovely old friend who gave me the

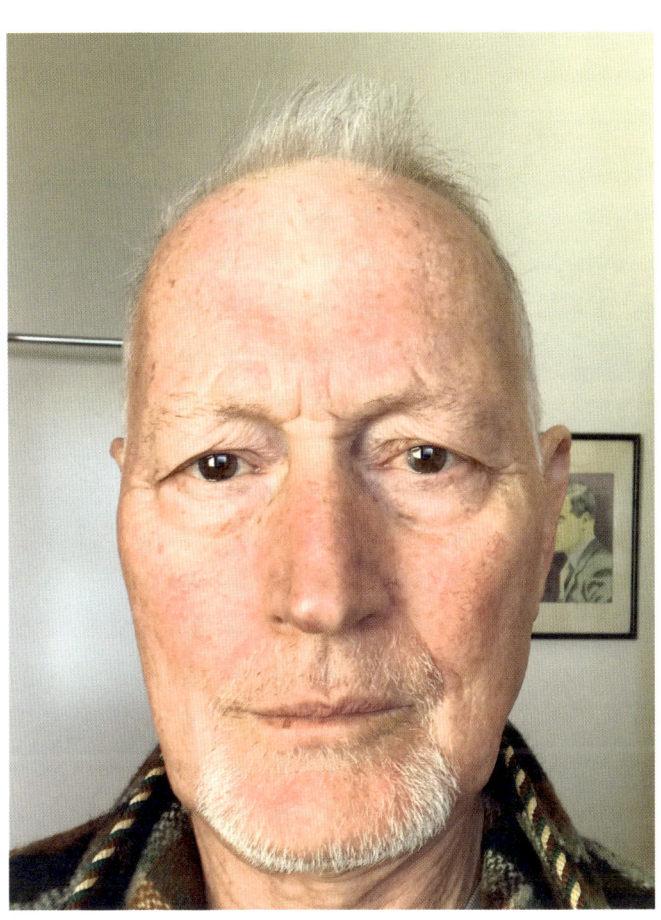

hugest – as he called it – *Hawke's Bay gin*. How Bess would have loved it.

Later:
A face with no eyebrows. My mother shaved hers off during the war years so she could draw on Marlene Dietrich-style pencilled-in eyebrows. It was when she was a tart. Her eyebrows never grew back. So all through her 'respectable' years as a mother and a matron she carried the signs of an earlier heresy. This is me without eyebrows (page 227). Second-to-last chemo on Monday. Strange when your face changes.

May 1, 1.43 a.m.

So begins one of the busiest times of my life (since I got sick). I go off to Welly on Thursday morning and at lunchtime do a gig at Unity Bookshop – that shop which is like a drawing room of intelligence, a fair space for the mind to find equipoise and sense and information. What an honour it is, a kind of intellectual version of *Dancing with the Stars*, wherein you take the stage and produce whatever moves you wish to make. I have prepared some readings and it's an honour to talk with Tilly about *Dear Oliver* in this space.

That same evening I head over to the City Gallery and *Little Queen* is shown, a film I made in the 1980s. It's many years since it came out. It was peopled by friends and family acting as a small crowd waiting to see the Queen drive by in 1954. I'll see the ghost of my mother, my father and friends when they

228

were younger, children who now have children themselves. *Little Queen* is such a strange tough film it will be a time travel in itself to see it.

Then next week I start heading into the huge edifice of the Auckland Writers Festival. I'm looking forward to this entertainment/inquisition with dear friend and excellent humane journalist David Herkt (himself an award-winning poet), who came to see me in my hospital room when I was in extremis. Anyone who can find you in Auckland Hospital is a friend well met.

I have my final blast of chemo in the week in between Wellington and the Festival, and I'm hoping I'll be over those almost crippling days of fatigue. I cannot complain. I am a writer and that is my calling. A writer needs to meet his or her own audience. I cannot just stay in my room alone. I need the warmth of an audience's breath. Besides, I want to find out what people think, their responses – what they want to know from the author of *Dear Oliver* but also that strangest of all documents, 'Hello Darkness'.

May 3, 1.35 p.m.

The most staggering thing happened to me in Wellington – I was presented with a $20,000 cheque as a prize/gift from the 50th Anniversary of Unity Books. The other recipient is Patricia Grace. I was so childishly overexcited, D and I ran as fast as our legs could carry us to Nikau and ordered a bracing bubbly.

The $20,000 cheque was given to Patricia Grace and myself for our writing, but also for a lifetime of social activism. All my adult life I have worked conscientiously for equality and improvement in the way we live, and I have never thought for a second of a reward. That's what makes this award so precious to me.

It was done with superb craft. I had finished doing my lunchtime gig and feeling at a low mental ebb when Tilly said they had an announcement to make about an award. It really only caught half my attention as I assumed it was some separate business. When she and Jo announced I was the winner of the Unity Books 50th Year Literary Award I was still struggling to catch up. I was given the envelope which I fancied carried a small card saying congratulations and perhaps a book token. When Tilly implored or rather ordered me to open it (it could have been Jo, my consciousness was still on catch-up) I saw a cheque, and then I saw the figure $20,000. My eyes then checked the written words as it seemed so unreal. It was at this point I became aware I had not only been given a great gift but I had also been seduced into an artful game of complete and utter surprise. Nothing in my entire life surprised me more.

I have often thought of the other side of the coin: and this is the life of all artists – disappointment at not winning a prize, hurt at being passed over in awards. The dark resentments going back to childhood, a seething black blood of rage. We have all experienced this demoralising and destructive mood. It eats into the soul and sours all that is good.

Yet here was I crowing about my good luck, knowing other writers are equally as likely to have won that wonderful award. I can think of four or five others very easily. How do they feel? And shouldn't I pipe down and just be grateful?

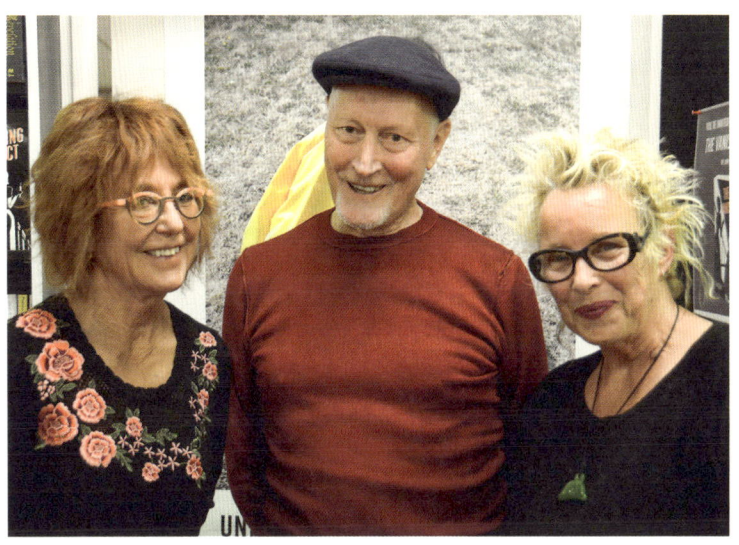

Winning as against losing is such a false dynamic. The very words are punishing. (Who doesn't secretly in their heart feel they're a loser?) And winning raises you on to an unreal plateau, as if the work you do has magically changed from what it was the second before.

But I have to confess to feeling all day as if I were glowing with happiness, as if I had actually been confirmed as being valuable in the arts/writing community – that I was 'somebody' (as against the nothingness of my secret self). I asked myself if I was given this prize because I had cancer. I did hope it wasn't, as my cancer has not changed anything, though it has led me into a wider and deeper public communication with 'Hello Darkness'. Had I revealed myself to people so they felt they knew me, a me which to myself is variable, hardly transparent, yet a self I have spoken through with an almost rash ease? I couldn't answer that. The fact was, for whatever reason, I had been given that small old-fashioned oblong of paper on which was written, in ballpoint, the majesty of a gift.

Having banked the lovely lucre (telling myself it was to be saved for something special), I did find in David Jones an extremely beautiful Paul Smith leather satchel. I argued to myself it was something I would always have to remind me of a certain day in Wellington, frosty and bright, on which I was given the greatest – and most delightful – surprise of my life.

I have my final chemo session tomorrow.

Why am I so terrified before chemo? I mean on the day. I know I'm a nervous type. When I was a sprinter I was always waiting for the gun, then I'd be off. I'm in that kind of mood. Listening for the gun.

May 7, 5.28 a.m.

It was as I walked up the short number of stairs to the chemo clinic that I recalled that urgent night, seemingly so long ago, when D and I had come to this same place, to see the radiology specialist. She had remained behind after work especially to see me. I had no idea what was happening. We were coming to see a specialist, I knew that. But I had reached such an abstract state of pain that nothing seemed quite real. We went into her office. But let me explain. There are specialists with faces like masks, faces afraid to divulge emotion. Others like my radiologist are entirely human and I could see, glancing into her face, empathy, understanding, sense. Yet such was the isolation of my pain I could read the signs but they meant very little to me. We talked – about what I am no longer sure. But I do remember this: she said, 'You are in a lot of pain, I want you to go into hospital.' Before this she had looked through my symptoms on screen. As I have said elsewhere, they were coloured fiery flares, as if we were in a plane bombing Dresden and far below there were these incendiary explosions. All else was black and white. Even I understood that those flares were my cancer.

This was really the beginning of my hospitalisation for what my oncologist today called my 'aggressive cancer'. I felt a curious relief to hear this. So many months later (six) I had reached a point where I doubted I had ever really been that sick. Was it my queer proclivity towards self-dramatisation? Was my cancer in fact never really life-threatening? This is what I thought now that I could walk without a stick (mostly), was no longer bowed with pain and had become the poster boy for recovery. As we walked into the clinic there were others on crutches now, and I nodded to them gracious as a queen. I could walk unaided. I had gone through all the radiation, hormone treatment and chemotherapy they could throw at me. It was my last chemo. Was it possible to feel almost sentimental about it?

The elderly cadaverous man beside me had had his grandson go and fetch a pie from the caf (mushroom and chicken, the grandson recommended). There were voices over the divide that were at the level of people talking in an airport (about a visit to Brussels). There was a discreet bustle of nurses attending to others in the clinic. It was a golden standard that no one was tragic. Everyone was upbeat, a little like people attending a funeral and making over-animated small talk while we waited for the main action to begin.

So this was the end of my chemo treatment. The oncologist had told me what was to follow. Four hormone tablets a day – Zytiga – to be taken on an empty stomach. They are meant to be as effective as chemo, though it appears there is no absolute science proving it. I felt curiously free.

The kindly oncologist warned me that I might feel flat. The great challenge of chemo was over. What was I facing now?

She was right of course. I had sharpened my resistance to overcome the challenge of chemo. I had lost most of my hair; my eyebrows had gone fugitive; I was the weight I was when I was in my twenties. Without my clothes I was skeletal, with an ugly belt of flesh above my hips which came from the Prednisone. But the fact was I was alive, I could walk, my cancer had been challenged, called to a halt – be it momentary or permanent, nobody knows. I could live with this impermanence: it was so much better than what I had been offered before. Now that long-ago night visiting the radiology specialist seemed like a dream. I was freed into living my own life again. It was, to some extent, a diminished life yet it was also a life expanded in consciousness. I could not unknow: I could comprehend, understand and move forward. It was my last chemo. With luck I might never come back.

Down to Daybreak

'*Darkness honestly lived through is a place of wonder and life*' – Robert Lowell

My days now seem calmer, less eventful. I'm far away from the sense of deep crisis which so marked these pages. Yet I'm reminded, too, of the provisional nature of my health with each small incoming crisis. (A question of bone density, further crumbling of bone in my back.) I've come to realise there is no 'remission' as such – rather, a suspended state of an indelicate being. I congratulate the doctors on delivering me to this state of intermediate health, but its provisional nature also tells me I should enjoy it to the full. I'm aware of the cost, and the costs. I'm like someone who has escaped something grave and from now on draws a deep gulp of breath. I'll always be amazed to be alive.

When I look back I see the recent past as a remarkable efflorescence, a time when I came vividly awake, as it were, to the true lineaments of my life: what was important, what did the past mean, what is the shape of my future?

You could say my relationship to life – as to death – is the secret or hidden pivot of this whole book. (At one point I wrote that the writing was 'a form of inquiry into how one conducts one's life or equally one's death'.) Yet again and again in these postings I talked of luck. Not bad luck, as it should have been, but a feeling of luckiness. I can't specifically say where this feeling came from. Was it a sense of the deepened love between me and my partner, Douglas? We drew closer together and I felt his care for me, his love for me. Who couldn't respond to this great gift? My being sick had thrust me into an almost abject state of dependence. Douglas's silent caring for me, guarding me, looking out for me – this quietly astonished me, then it settled into the core of my being as a statement of his great love. Now we spent nearly every minute in every hour together. We were together. There was no questioning it. I understood my own dependence on him, but also my deep love for him and his equally strong abiding love for me. Would we have discovered this without the sickness? I don't know but I doubt it. Any grave illness is a great test, and a mortal illness is a greater test still. What can I say? We discovered that we loved one another in the shade of death. It's that simple. That was why I felt so lucky.

But it wasn't only this. I began to see daily life itself was a form of a gift – just to be alive was a prescient thing. Of course I had many bad days but I also had this constant almost shrill sense of astonishment at just being alive. I had got so close to the edge of death in those early days in hospital. I had breathed in its rank air, I sensed its presence. In terms of that, I felt lucky just to be ambulant. I even felt lucky to have a few years left – if it is years. I did not and do not know.

Now I am in this ambiguous space of quietude. I gather my cancer has been momentarily beaten into submission. When the stoic urologist – a man with a face used to giving bad news – said to me in the early days 'We're going to throw everything at it', I accepted this numbly. What else could I do? I knew almost nothing. (As I have said, at no point did any specialist or doctor sit me down, describe my diagnosis in words I could understand, or give me a clear prognosis.) I had to gather my situation from the few sentences the urologist told me, or whatever research I could do on the arcane sheets of information given to me, much as a travel agent, clear in his mind as to your destination, hands out a ticket along with the small print as to Acts of God and loss of luggage. But these really amounted to guesses. If anything, I worked out my predicament from the gravity with which the specialists treated me. I knew the cancer had entered the bones of my back, near the spinal column and that some of the bones were crumbling. From this I knew my situation was dire.

I was not one of those men who threw himself into a frenzy of research to 'control' the disease. Implicitly I trusted the urologist who initially gave me the bad news. The oncologist herself described the cancer as 'aggressive', so the treatment deployed radiation, hormone therapy and chemotherapy all at the same time – and its outcome, in the end, was definite: the shrinking of the tumours by half. I was, however, not initially sure what this meant.

One evening my usual oncologist was away. I had a different oncologist so I took advantage of the situation to ask – bluntly – what does it mean? Tumours shrunken in half? She told me matter of factly that the cancer was now quiescent and would be tracked by monthly tests, and in time we would know whether, if the cancer came back, it was mild or virulent. I gathered from this I was in a suspended state. I was not cured – of course. There is no cure, I knew that from the beginning. But I was being given the chance to recommence life. To live as if I did not have cancer. Or rather, to live with the condition that the cancer could effloresce at some later stage. As to the present, I could live as if it no longer existed inside me.

If you have lived under the guillotine, living with a sharp knife is infinitely preferable.

What had I learned? Someone returned from a far-away place is meant to return with news. My news, I am afraid, is rather banal. The worth of small things. As my horizon shrank, so the surroundings grew more significant. I just liked being alive. Something like a morning coffee in a cafe became an acme of pleasure – as thrilling as going to the circus as a child. I had less energy. I found it difficult to walk far. I still had trouble with my breathing which was shallow and painful. Yet I was alive. I always come back to this fact.

And I have to confess that the intimacy of FB helped me stay in good spirits. It was a kind of living community, contrarily delivered digitally and in the absence of any human touch. I got to like this absence of human touch. I liked the ethereality of it and the absence of messy actual real-time contact. That's a terrible confession to make. (It gave my poor old body space in which to ruminate and move about slowly. I didn't have energy for meetings and, in fact, when quite close friends got in touch and asked to meet, as often as not I evaded them.)

Yet on line I had an enormous effulgence of energy to respond, say hi, affirm, acknowledge. Did it mean anything? Yes, it did. Happening in real time I was offered comfort, support, sympathy, empathy. These are not small things. In fact they are enormous things. They helped me. They salved me of isolation and loneliness. Often they removed self-doubt. I felt I was watched, even watched over. This seems a strange thing to say of a digital presence, yet it is true.

But here is another terrible confession. At times I wasn't sure I was fortunate to have such a dramatic complaint. Life had ceased to be boring. I always had something happening. People poured their concentration on me. People showed their concern, friends their love. How different it was from everyday life where you struggled against anomie, against a sense you were unimportant and that time itself was a fixative to which you were glued, incapable of movement or even registering your presence. I know this is being absurd, but I became used to being cherished and cared for. I wasn't so much selfish as relishing what the disease had brought me. It wasn't like I was less selfish or incapable of envy: I had not magically become suffused with noble virtues; I was still the same incomplete individual, subject to envy and spite. But the sheer time element – of no longer having a normal life span – changed everything, condensed everything, filled what was an inherently vacant space with a charged meaning.

Was I being given a special pass? Yes, I was. I was excused from hard physical activities – nobody expected me to undertake normal household duties like sweeping a path after a storm. But there was also an expectation that the condensed time I was experiencing produced deeper thought. I am not sure that was so. The alternative was I had the strange leisure of nights without end, of days with no purpose in which to brood. Yet most often I had this noxious – was it a diseased? – cheerfulness. Was I actually thrilled to be mortally sick? Did this confer on me a specialness I had always sought? The fact was I had always wanted to be exceptional and this very ordinary disease now gave me my chance. Perhaps that was the secret behind my strange gloaming happiness: I was where I always wanted to be – loved, cherished, cared for, made special by my mortality.

This was childish, infantile, yet there is an element of truth to it. I had been rescued from the piercing isolation of everyday life and put at the centre of any number of concerns – the hospice, the oncologist, my doctor, Douglas, my FB friends. Sickness became an occupation, something to do: it defined me and, at long last, I could relax into the full condition of being wanted and looked after. This luxurious infantilism was one aspect of the sickness I have never really acknowledged. I became used to my exceptionalism. I did not want to return to the vast army of the ordinarily healthy – the unawake, you might say, unaware of when or where sickness might come, and who will then have to make sudden adjustments as to how to live life, see life – and see time and what time is doing to you. Of course time does not 'do anything to you'; it is your awareness of the brevity of time that changes everything: condenses, makes precious. I did not want to go back to that unspecified and vague sense that time existed as a kind of weight or oppression. I much preferred this sense of time as something precious. I liked experiencing time as vivid, as limited, almost a limited edition. I know this reveals a selfish persona. I refute the nobility of my condition and assert it is infused with as much selfishness and as many flaws as I had in ordinary life.

One gets to the core of the condition with the word mortal. It means human as against divine, according to the dictionary. I think these days we can drop the divine aspect: to be mortal means to be alive. But it also means – as in a mortal condition – to be facing death. An ordinary enough exceptionalism, really – more ordinary than you might think. (Besides there's a good chance now I might elude early death: I might live on till my eighties.) Alternatively, and this is something that terrifies me, the tumours on my spine and back may worsen and I might descend into a cauldron of unbearable pain and even immobility. This I cannot bear to think about.

But to come back to the core of my condition: it is or was of somebody facing death. It occurs to me the most remarkable outcome has been my ability to contemplate it and write about living with it. This has been the greatest gift. Every morning I awoke with the expectation I would be writing something about my daily experiences. During the time I was in hospital these were, as it were, front-line dispatches. As time went on the dispatches became more observational, more autobiographical. But how I loved the ease of communication, how I awoke each day with a sense of purpose. Was this a part of my strange joy too? To have a purpose is one of the greatest benefits a human can experience. So in the end it was the gift of all these words – my attempts to describe, evoke, limn my experience – that has been the unexpected side-effect of my mortality.

I'm aware of incompleteness and of my inability to describe fully the experience of cancer; but on a daily shuffling basis I've tried to describe the experience as it struck me. So this in the end is my confession: how I have loved writing, how I have attempted to evade mortality by putting my experiences into words, and how the creation of these words in themselves has been the greatest help to me. They have been my wheelchair, my walking stick, my drug and blanket: better, they have been precise words I have chosen.

And through FB I had the luxury of people listening. This is the inalienable other half of the situation. I wrote into a living circumstance to which people avidly responded. I was not existentially alone.

'It is in moments of illness that we are compelled to recognise that we live not alone but chained to a creature of a different kingdom, whole worlds apart, who has no knowledge of us and by whom it is impossible to make ourselves understood: our body'. That's Proust, in *Le Côté de Guermantes*.

I am chained to that body, it is true – one I am unsure is 'cured of cancer'. It's a fact: if I am unconvinced about my recovery, another side of me sings an oratorio to the fact I am excepted: within six months I have been pinged into a state of almost-health. I can walk. I can function. I am back inside my own thin skin. I am sentient and, as I write, I hear Douglas in the kitchen preparing a meal. We have friends coming by for dinner. The late afternoon is golden in its tinge. Ajax has caught a rat. My book, *Dear Oliver*, has been a success. I am putting together another book, this one. I am so lucky, so fucking Kylie Minogue lucky, that I really should pipe down and be silent. Accept that the future will take me where it may.

I decided to call this part of the book 'Down to Daybreak' because it really gives some sense of the optimism which gripped me even during the dark hours. This book exists to represent my experience with cancer. It is about a time when I faced what seemed the greatest crisis. At the very end of my posts I said I could not 'unknow' what I had learned. The fact is I do not want to unknow. I was given a strange gift, and I accepted it. I hope, in these pages, I have put it to good use.